W9-CEO-934

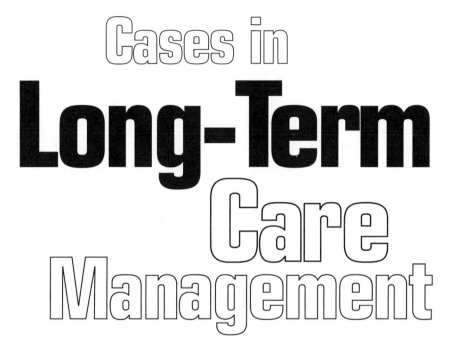

Volume II
Leadership Challenges in
Managing Change

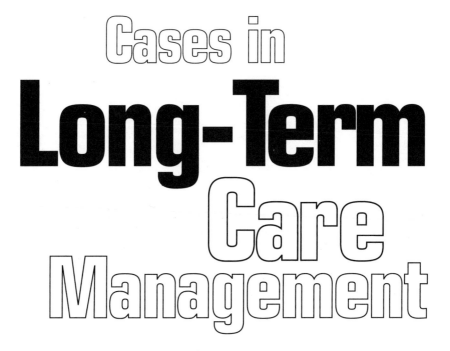

Cases in Long-Term Care Management

**Volume II
Leadership Challenges in
Managing Change**

Edited by
Donna Lind Infeld
John R. Kress

AUPHA Press/ Health Administration Press
Ann Arbor, Michigan 1995

99 98 97 96 95   5 4 3 2 1

LC: 89-060-374   ISBN 1-56793-033-6

The paper used in this publication meets the minimum requirements of American National Standard for Information Sciences—Permanence of Paper for Printed Library Materials, ANSI Z39.48-1984. ∞™

Health Administration Press
A division of the Foundation
   of the American College of
   Healthcare Executives
1021 East Huron Street
Ann Arbor, Michigan 48104
(313) 764-1380

Association of University Programs
   in Health Administration
1911 North Fort Myer Drive, Suite 503
Arlington, VA 22209
(703) 524-5500

To Marcel, the light of my life—DLI.

To Madeline, John, Anna, and Steve, who blessed us that we might be a blessing—JRK.

Contents

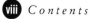

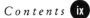
- Developing facility policy
- Conflict over information between family and OBRA
- OBRA protection of residents' rights

- New nursing home ethics committee
- Advance directives
- Conflict among family, physician, staff, and resident

Part IV Operations Challenges

- Care coordination
- Team leadership
- Socialization and conflict

- Care for HIV/AIDS patients
- Ethical decision making
- Human resources issues

- Staff dissatisfaction and turnover
- Impact on quality of care
- Survey deficiencies

- Relationship between hospital and subacute unit
- Disaster policy
- The Los Angeles earthquake

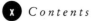

Part V   Human Resources and Labor Relations

Part VI   Program and Financial Development

Part VII   Strategic Planning and Marketing

Foreword

FIVE YEARS ago the Association of University Programs in Health Administration (AUPHA) published *Cases in Long-Term Care Management: Building the Continuum*. The practice landscape has changed dramatically since then, and health care reform, incremental, rather than immediate and sudden, is well on the way toward assuring the incorporation of long-term care within a more seamless, human, and efficient general system of care. The challenges for administrators managing in a rapidly and constantly changing long-term care environment under intense scrutiny will only increase as we enter the new century.

This volume represents a maturation of the relationship between the practitioner and the academic community. Virtually all of the cases included reflect the growing collaboration between health administration programs, their faculty, and the community of practitioners and managers. The geometric expansion of organizationally integrated health care services requires all health care managers to understand and master the unique environment within which long-term managers must operate. The first of these volumes demonstrated the potential of higher education to help the long-term care community build administrative strength; this collection recognizes the contributions of the long-term care community in improving the educational experience and knowledge of our students, so that they will effectively manage a more complex health care system now and in the future.

We remain indebted to the seminal support eight years ago of The Robert Wood Johnson Foundation, which rekindled (or provoked) the interest of our faculty in long-term care. The long-term care industry has become an important player in improving the quality of health for our communities. As the public member for the Board for Nursing Home Administrators for the Commonwealth of Virginia, I can only applaud the continued effort of the long-term health care practitioner and academic communities to improve the quality of the educational experiences of its managers.

Henry A. Fernandez, J.D.
President and Chief Executive Officer
Association of University Programs
 in Health Administration
Arlington, Virginia

Introduction: Leadership Development and the Use of Management Case Studies in Long-Term Care Administration

The Need for Leadership Development

THE AGING population in the United States and Canada is a dynamic force altering the face of health and human services delivery systems. Stresses generated by the increasing number of elderly persons and other population groups needing long-term care services tax these systems, stimulating new service structures, reimbursement mechanisms, and relationships among providers. Demand from the many organizations in the field for creative and effective executive leadership is growing dramatically.

The turn of the twenty-first century is a particularly challenging time for nursing home administrators. Implementation of the many and complex provisions of the Omnibus Reconciliation Act of 1987 places new demands on administrators and staff throughout nursing facilities. The Patient Self-Determination Act, passed as part of the Omnibus Reconciliation Act of 1990, is another example of the external changes necessitating new responses in nursing facilities. In addition, tools new to the long-term care environment, such as total quality management (TQM) and continuous quality improvement (CQI), change relationships among staff members and between staff and management, and also place new demands for data collection and monitoring. These are but a few examples of the dramatic developments currently taking place in the provision of quality long-term care services.

Adapted from Infeld, D. L., and J. R. Kress 1989. *Cases in Long-Term Care Management: Building the Continuum.* Owings Mills, MD: AUPHA Press.

Recent growth in the number and complexity of long-term care service organizations has been dramatic, and projections for future expansion are even greater. In spite of the expanding need for skilled long-term care administrators, most health administration program graduates continue to be drawn to management practice in other settings. However, many factors previously perceived as deterrents to health care administrators gravitating toward the field of long-term care management now are changing. The professional image of the long-term care administrator is steadily improving. Salary incentives and benefit package levels have become more attractive. As organizations increase in size and complexity, so do administrative opportunities. The demand for executives with the sensitivities, experience, and expertise required in long-term care services also is increasing in various health, housing, insurance, and related organizations as vertical integration and service diversification continues. The challenges involved in care for the chronically ill require administrators with a firm grounding in management and strong executive leadership skills. Administrators must be effective managers to survive in this demanding arena.

Providing long-term care services offers qualified managers and administrators unique rewards, poses unique problems, and demands unique management skills. Administrators must appreciate, understand, and adapt to this uniqueness. The profession necessitates blending management and client interests. Meeting client needs and dealing with family and community scrutiny is considerably more demanding in long-term care than in other settings. The constantly changing, fragmented system of health, housing, and social services, and the bewildering array of financing and reimbursement systems demands leadership and creativity in building and orchestrating the seamless continuum of long-term care services we all desire for our elders.

Further, the intensity of services offered in nonacute settings is expanding rapidly. For example, many nursing facilities now deliver highly sophisticated subacute care and rehabilitation that until recently was provided only in hospitals. Terminal care also is increasingly being provided in long-term care facilities.

Long-term care administrators face considerably different staffing patterns than do other health care administrators. Nursing home directors must recruit, retain, motivate, and maintain quality personnel in the face of shortages of nurses and other professionals and high turnover of support staff, who often work in extremely stressful environments. Generally, these directors work with fewer levels of management and professional staff than do their hospital counterparts.

The general knowledge areas required to manage long-term care facilities and systems encompass service coordination, clinical knowledge, social and community factors, law, ethics, management theory, supervision, system design, and real estate, among others. Specialty knowledge areas include chronicity and its implications, geriatric assessment and care, characteristics of specific service settings, and family relations. Necessary administrative skills include the management of finances, human resources, information systems, and complex systems arrangements. Thus, long-term care administration requires multiple levels of knowledge for effective management. It also requires considerable patience to deal with continuous changes resulting from being the most heavily regulated segment of health services.

Providing long-term care is a management business; it is also a people business. Administrators need to manage an array of services for long-term care populations. The field needs executives who are disciplined, know how to manage, and are sensitive to the needs of clients, families, and staff. They must be able to cross service lines and break traditional barriers to offer a wide range of services, including, for example, housing and child day care. A long-term care administrator is increasingly likely to work in an organizational structure that includes multiple service levels. Leading the development of client-centered care at these various levels is one of the most important challenges in health care today.

The Use of Management Case Studies

Earthquake! Union action! Life and death decisions! Competitive threats! Financial collapse!

Decision making is the major function of executives. In challenging situations administrators must lead, but how do they learn to make good decisions? One way is to practice. The use of management case studies has proven to be an effective device for gaining decision making experience in an educational environment. While in the real world there seldom is a chance to experiment or try again, working with case studies allows various strategies to be tried and errors to be corrected and forgiven. The case method has been used for management education in university programs for many years, and it also has been successfully employed by industry in executive development and continuing education programs.

What is a Case?

The term "case" is used in many ways, e.g., patient case, law case. This book presents *management cases*, cases that describe a situation or problem faced by an administrator that require analysis, planning a course of action, and decision making. The cases are designed to provide sufficient background information for students and readers to understand the complex environments in which management problems occur, consider various options, and recommend a strategy or strategies to solve the problems. It is important to note that the actions portrayed in the cases do not necessarily represent good management or wise decisions. Students and instructors should determine the appropriateness of the performance portrayed and identify alternative courses of action that could or should have been taken.

Purposes of the Book

The goal of this book is to present a range of cases which can assist students and readers in developing or improving on general awareness of facility-based, long-term care management techniques, analytical skills, professional judgement, personal values, and communication skills. In particular, the following professional faculties will be addressed and considered:

Knowledge. The cases present information about policies and pro- cedures, roles and responsibilities of staff, and characteristics of clients who use services. Cases are not necessarily the most efficient way to gain factual knowledge about programs for facilities, rather, they serve as an integrating vehicle for the aggregate of knowledge gained through ex- perience, previous reading, and course work. Situations and information presented in the cases should result in a synthesis of experience with concepts and theories. Studying the coherent whole also will expand and enrich understanding of theoretical ideas and approaches.

Management techniques. Cases provide the opportunity to apply tech- niques such as forecasting, budgeting, staffing, and strategic planning to specific situations. The methods used by principals in these cases may be appropriate or inappropriate; readers should evaluate the techniques used and apply others to the cases if they are thought to be more effective. In the case study method, deciding when to use a particular technique is as important as knowing how to use it.

Analytical skills. Clear thinking, problem clarification, and sound decision making are extremely difficult skills to teach. A major benefit of the case study method is that it directly helps students to develop each of them. Cases simulate complex and ambiguous situations faced by administrators involving insufficient information, conflicting pressures, and lacking any "absolutely right" solution. These situations do require that some decision be made, possibly the decision to take no action at all. After applying appropriate analytical techniques to the situation, readers must combine information, theoretical concepts, and common sense into a systematic process in order to develop plans and a strategy for how to proceed.

Professional judgment. Optimal decisions require good judgment. It is essential to review all sides of an issue, to minimize emotional reactions in the decision-making process, and to reach decisions benefiting both clients and the organization. Professional administrators are distinguished by their ability to do this well. Again, that it allows opportunities to practice sound decision making is a strength of the case study method of learning.

Personal values. Values are learned early in life and are difficult to change. Their influence and impact become apparent in examining the decision-making processes used in case situations. Organizational problem solving involves confronting the basis for and implications of possible decisions, projecting expected consequences, and weighing potential risks. In practice, managers rarely face "win-win" situations. Through case study decision making, readers can assess the values and priorities governing their actual decision making. Cases test the validity of personal values and provide opportunities to examine their consequences for executive decisions.

Case studies also provide an excellent vehicle for building *communication skills*. Using both formal and informal presentations, including role playing, they provide experience in public speaking, quick thinking, and defending an analysis and resulting position. These are essential competencies for successful administrators. In formal educational programs, cases can be used to diagnose weaknesses and to help develop new skills. In the corporate environment, cases can be used to sharpen abilities, expand perspectives, and reinforce corporate culture.

How to Use the Cases

This case book is designed for use principally by two audiences: students in formal educational programs and executives in continuing education or training programs. In formal educational settings it can be used with upper level undergraduate or graduate students in health services administration, public health, gerontology, business, and nursing programs. The cases can be used in long-term care courses, in general health administration courses to provide long-term care material, or in "capstone" case studies courses. Within the practice community, it can be used by long-term care organizations and corporations in executive development and continuing education programs.

Cases can be used in lectures as reference points or examples, or students and readers can be required to analyze cases independently or in groups. In analysis or role playing situations, participants can take the perspective of the administrator or management consultants brought in to recommend optimal courses of action. Alternatively, participants can take roles representing the range of actors and interested audiences involved in the case. Learning with case studies is *active* learning. Participants must be prepared to get involved, feel what the administrator in each case is feeling, and examine how other participants might react.

Case analysis can take various forms. Basic steps in any analysis include:

1. Selecting a role or perspective from which to analyze the case
2. Analyzing the case—prioritizing relevant issues and players, essential internal and external facts, assumptions fundamental to the analysis, and identifying missing information
3. Identifying problems—what is the fundamental problem or issue, which are underlying, and are they controllable?
4. Considering alternative courses of action—evaluating the strengths and weaknesses of each option and prioritizing.
5. Deciding how to proceed—justifying the decision and assessing the feasibility of its implementation
6. Considering operational implications—developing timetables and assigning responsibility for the completion of tasks.

There are no right answers to the problems presented in these cases. However, some strategies will tend to be more promising than others. The important point is that a thorough analysis of the specific circumstances of the case is necessary in order to identify optimum recommendations. All six stages of the analytical process are critical to its successful implementation.

Cases in this Book

These cases were written to present an introduction to a range of long-term care facility settings and to portray a variety of administrative problems and situations commonly encountered by their executives. Settings include nursing facilities providing subacute, skilled, intermediate and special care, continuing care retirement communities, hospitals, residential care for the mentally retarded, and vertically integrated health care organizations. The key decision maker generally is the administrator or chief executive officer. Other important managers include assistant administrators, directors of nursing, social services, and other departments, and long-term care consultants.

Most of these cases were prepared by faculty members from member programs of the Association of University Programs in Health Administration, in collaboration with practicing long-term care administrators. Some cases use the name of the facility and actual data. Others mask the organizational identity, yet the facts presented are based on true experiences and situations. A footnote to each case indicates their factual basis.

Some issues the cases address affect most long-term care facilities, including problems of staff turnover and recruitment, quality of care, reimbursement, and strategic planning. Other issues are more specific to individual setting characteristics, such as unionized or potentially unionized facilities. Each case reveals both general and specific issues. While it is impossible to present all possible situations that might confront long-term care administrators, this collection presents a diverse array of current issues and problems. It provides a sense of the variety of activities and problems which are part of this challenging career.

The book's 23 cases are organized by having been clustered into broad topical areas, which are identified in the table of contents. The Integrative Framework (Table 1) provides a clearer picture of the range of issues addressed by each case. A separate volume, the *Teaching Notes for Cases in Long-Term Care Management*, provides additional guidance to help instructors in selecting cases related to specific topic areas. The *Teaching Notes* for each case include a brief case summary, a statement of objectives, background information, problems and issues raised by the case, description of background expected of participants, and approaches to analysis of the case. Some notes additionally have a section describing how the situation actually was resolved. The *Teaching Notes* frequently also include material that can be distributed during case discussion.

Conclusion

The variety of services and the issues faced by the administrators featured in these cases highlight important management challenges in long-term care facility administration. Strong and creative executive leadership for these types of diverse organizations is vital if new strategies are to improve care quality within an environment of severe fiscal, staffing, and other resource constraints.

Table 1 Integrative Framework of Case Content Areas

Case	I OBRA	II Quality	III Ethics	IV Operation	V HR	VI Finance	VII Planning	Physical Plant	Survey	Case Mgmt.	Spec'l Pops.
Community Care	X			Board		Data					
Ridgecrest	MDS	X		X	X	X				X	
United Hebrew	X		X								
The Fenway		X		X					X		
Whispering Pines		TQM/CQI		Corp	X						
Westmount		TQM/CQI		Corp	Union						
Rockingham			X	Board							
Jewish Homes	X		X	Board							
Marlton			X	X							Subacute
Good Shepherd				Board	X					X	
Lockwood			X		X		X				AIDS
The Commons		X		X	X			X	X		
Holy Cross				X				X			
Chapel Square		X		X	X		X				Subacute
Jennett Manor				Corp	Union				X		
Westview				X	Union						
Clark				Board		Capital	X	X			
ConstantCaring	X	X		Corp	TEFRA	X	Market				
Riverview		X		X	X	X	X		X	X	
NE Health Sys				X			X		X		
Ocean Point				X		Data	X	X			MR/DD
Kidron Bethel				Board		Data	X				
Angel Crest			Values	Board	X	X	X	X			

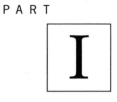
OBRA Implementation

Community Care Center: Leadership Crisis at a Public Nursing Facility

Robert H. Daugherty, Keith Boles, and James A. Irvin

I: Background

The Organization

COMMUNITY CARE CENTER (CCC) is a 120-bed nursing home located in a community of 70,000 persons. The facility was built as a county residential home for indigent elderly. It was redesignated a nursing home in the early 1970s when funding for the care of the elderly became available under Medicare and Medicaid. The county encouraged the formation of a not-for-profit 501(c)3 corporation, Community Care Center, Inc. (CCC). The facility was leased to CCC, with the county maintaining ownership of the building and grounds. Construction of the 60-bed facility was funded through bonds and taxation. CCC's 20-year lease required a nominal payment of $1 per year. In return, it agreed to accept all residents, regardless of their ability to pay.

In 1981, CCC, again through county taxing Authority, built an additional 60 beds. At that point, the county and CCC entered into another lease agreement throughout the term of that CCC would make lease payments of $11,000 per month.

The Facility

The original 60-bed facility was adequate for its time. The 60-bed addition was constructed as a second floor, but due to budget constraints, had been poorly designed. Although it met basic code requirements, there was insufficient common space for residents, traffic flow was poor, and there were too few windows. The resulting facility was overly institutional, dark, and unattractive. No renovation has been done since the addition was built with the exception of a porch and lounge area that was added two years ago with funds raised by the auxiliary.

Since the late 1980s the nursing home has placed difficult medical and behavioral residents on the second floor. This has resulted in an image of the second floor as a "dumping ground," and new residents generally did not want to be placed there. Consequently, the first floor remained full while the second floor often had beds available, but was avoided by prospective residents, who preferred to wait for an opening on the first floor.

Governance

Community Care Center has a self-perpetuating board of nine directors, in accordance with its articles of incorporation and bylaws. Board members serve staggered three-year terms with three new members being appointed each year. There is no limitation on how long a board member may serve. Three current members have been on the board since their original appointments over 15 years ago.

Since its founding, the board has attempted to maintain a balanced membership, including persons from health and welfare professions and agencies, the business community, the university, and at least one member from the southern area of the county and one from the northern area. In addition, the bylaws require that a member of the county commission be a regular, voting member.

The philosophy that was embodied in the original charter provided guidance and continuity for CCC. The articles of incorporation contain the statement of purpose, which has remained unchanged:

> To manage, operate and promote a retirement center or nursing home for the aged on a not-for-profit basis for the benefit of the needy people of the county; and to cooperate with and assist the county commission and provide for the indigent and elderly in accordance with the county's responsibility.

The three original board members, who were loyal to the administrator, felt the mission of the organization required that the facility not operate at a profit. They were not in the least concerned about its financial situation and believed the administrator was performing according to expectations.

Throughout the 1980s, new board members periodically attempted to raise issues about the administration and financial management of the facility, but their efforts were generally ignored by the administrator, and lacked support from others on the board.

The board traditionally met once a month. It had no functioning committees other than the executive committee composed of the officers and the county commissioner. All of the work was done at monthly meetings; materials were prepared and distributed to members, usually during the meeting itself.

The board delegated all power and authority for operations to the administrator, and typically did not intervene in staff or operational matters. The only exception to this rule was an ongoing concern about resident food. In the 1980s, several board members became aware of complaints from residents and their families concerning the dietary service. This issue was addressed at several board meetings and continuing assurances were made that something would be done, but the complaints persisted. Finally, the administrator hired a full-time dietician, but still the complaints continued. The issue came to a head at a board meeting during which the new dietician, who had been invited to attend, and three board members engaged in a heated debate. Everyone agreed the issue had gotten out of hand; the board members backed off and the food service did seem to improve somewhat, although sporadic complaints continued. Within a year complaints began to increase again. The board periodically discussed plans for the future, but its overall operational mode was to respond to current issues and take its lead from the administrator. This modus operandi often led to unsatisfactory results.

Some board members felt frustrated at this pattern of having insufficient information for making well-informed decisions and that the administrator had not exerted the leadership and support they felt was needed. The general feeling of board members, however, has been that running a nursing home is a thankless endeavor, misunderstood by the public, and overly regulated by the government. They thought the administrator was doing an adequate job; nursing home administration is a calling, rather than a profession, and, therefore, that finding a replacement would have been difficult.

The board's annual evaluation of the administrator followed a format whereby the administrator left the room and the board discussed his performance and salary increase. When the administrator returned the board would indicate how much of a salary increase it was granting and would then make some general statements about the nice job he was doing.

Executive Management

The administrator, Mr. Dolinsky, had been with CCC since its inception and was the only administrator it had ever had. He had a baccalaureate degree when he was hired, and has since earned an undergraduate degree in health administration. Mr. Dolinsky has been active in state and national nursing home associations and is generally well-regarded by his peers.

His leadership style is to fully delegate responsibility for day-to-day operations. He has, however, maintained personal control of financial matters. He avoids discussing issues or problems with the board unless someone else brings them up, and then provides only limited information. He seldom offers suggestions and, more often than not, his comments center around why something cannot be done.

Nursing facility reform contained in the Omnibus Budget Reconciliation Act of 1987 (OBRA), in Mr. Dolinsky's view, is a nightmare of additional federal requirements put upon nursing homes, necessitating additional staffing and resources which the government is not willing to fund. He saw no problem with the way things were prior to OBRA's inception.

Mr. Dolinsky tends to be rather indirect and non-supportive with subordinates. He has placed people in positions and then has assumed they were performing unless he heard complaints or they brought problems to him. When problems were brought to his attention he seldom has done anything about them, so the staff has learned to either ignore them or solve them on their own. He has assumed department heads knew what he thought of them so there was no need for formal performance appraisals.

The director of nursing, Ms. Babcock, had been with the facility for over 15 years, and administered the nursing care services with an iron hand. The nursing staff feared her. Her modus operandi at staff meetings was to maintain a list of complaints against other department heads. If the meeting turned to problems in nursing, Ms. Babcock would recite a litany of problems in other areas. This generally succeeded in deflecting attention from nursing problems and reduced most staff meetings to exchanges of noncontroversial information.

Service

The facility had provided acceptable service over the years, its reputation maintained by its image as a community resource that would accept everyone, and its caring core staff. This core group represented about 20 percent of the employees; the rest of the staff tended to turn over every year.

Recently, its policy to accept all applicants led CCC to admit some residents it was not equipped to handle. These residents were almost always placed on the second floor, with the quality of their care varying dramatically. Prior to OBRA '87, quality problems generally went undetected in state surveys, which were concerned primarily with paper compliance. When deficiencies were cited, the administrator typically responded with a perfunctory plan of correction which was usually accepted by the state, but never monitored. Residents and their families complained from time to time, but complaints generally went unheeded.

The one truly bright spot of CCC operations was the auxiliary, a group of dedicated women from the community who, led by a member of the CCC Board of Directors, came in weekly to operate the beauty shop and other activities for the residents. The auxiliary also was instrumental in raising thousands of dollars over the years and generating goodwill from the community.

Nursing care followed the medical model with limited social services or activities available other than bingo, chapel services, and occasional special programs. Services were based on the state's nursing home guidelines, and only the administrator and director of nurses were aware of their requirements.

The Board of Directors was not informed of the annual state survey and its requirements, nor had it seen a survey report. The administrator generally treated the annual inspection as a minor event and included its occurrence in his administrator's report briefly, without dwelling on its content.

Finance

Over the years the Board of Directors paid little systematic attention to financial matters other than to adopt the annual budget and review financial reports, including the annual audit. The administrator prepared a budget, but it usually was adopted with little discussion, and generally was ignored during the year. Included in the annual audit was a cursory ritual whereby the audit firm came to a board meeting and presented noncontroversial findings, which were quickly approved.

The facility consistently had its operating deficits underwritten by the county (see Table 1.1). In fact, the county and the board treated CCC very much as a de facto department of the county, in which the facility presented its budget to the county commission and the county allocated funds to subsidize operating losses. There were many board members who felt that for the facility to break even or make money operationally meant their charges would be excessive or they would not be accepting sufficiently needy clients.

In 1986–87 the facility purchased a financial software package, but not until 1990 did it hire a person with some computer background who

Table 1.1 Community Care Center Statement of Revenues and Expenses Last Five Years

	5 Years Ago	4 Years Ago	3 Years Ago	2 Years Ago	Last Year
Patient Service Revenues	$2,112,290	$2,128,627	$2,335,312	$2,523,115	$2,506,516
Contractual Adjustment	$0	$0	$0	$0	$0
(Medicaid retroactive settlements for prior years)	$2,112,290	$2,128,627	$2,335,312	$2,523,115	$2,506,516
Other operating revenue	$35,030	$41,327	$25,596	$113,504	$103,325
	$2,147,320	$2,169,954	$2,360,908	$2,636,619	$2,609,841
Operating Expenses					
Nursing services	$867,332	$1,012,535	$1,122,317	$1,260,182	$1,505,390
Other professional service					
Dietary	$350,233	$374,757	$393,274	$456,493	$536,455
Laundry	$59,071	$63,841	$79,317	$88,919	$81,412
Housekeeping	$144,441	$163,188	$188,240	$211,778	$221,616
Plant operations	$339,933	$323,834	$354,018	$375,263	$370,119
General and administrative	$490,615	$285,398	$304,975	$297,915	$303,796
	$2,251,625	$2,223,553	$2,442,141	$2,690,550	$3,018,788
Operating Revenue Over (Under) Operating Expenses	($104,305)	($53,599)	($81,233)	($53,931)	($408,947)
Nonoperating Revenues					
Tax appropriation	$0	$0	$100,000	$0	$0
Forgiveness lease	$0	$0	$0	$0	$224,000
Investment income	$13,466	$15,825	$21,783	$20,447	$8,304
	$13,466	$15,825	$121,783	$20,447	$232,304
Revenues Over (Under) Expenses	($90,839)	($37,774)	$40,550	($33,484)	($176,643)

could use it. Even then CCC did not use its entire capabilities, and opted for a hybrid of hand-generated and computerized reports.

Administrative costs for the facility were almost twice the average for facilities across the state. Tables 1.2 and 1.3 contain balance sheets and operating statements for the last five years. Table 1.4 is a plan for staffing full-time equivalents.

Table 1.2 Community Care Center Balance Sheets Last Five Years

	5 Years Ago	4 Years Ago	3 Years Ago	2 Years Ago	Last Year
Current Assets					
Cash	$147,025	$227,223	$175,995	$102,316	$48,202
Repurchase agreement					
Accounts receivable					
Patients	$241,337	$263,290	$285,337	$243,762	$211,800
County	$0	$0	$0	$0	$0
Medicaid voluntary					
contribution	$0	$0	$0	$175,420	$0
Prepaid supplies	$2,173	$2,173	$2,173	$2,173	$1,086
Prepaid expense	$19,587	$34,628	$30,719	$39,465	$18,424
Total current assets	$410,122	$527,314	$494,224	$563,136	$279,512
Assets limited use	$0	$0	$56,000	$93,095	$34,206
Property and equipment					
Land and					
improvements	$174,800	$179,800	$180,980	$180,980	$180,980
Building	$1,097,956	$1,105,629	$1,133,271	$1,157,322	$1,280,854
Building addition	$905,654	$905,654	$905,654	$905,654	$905,654
Equipment	$294,210	$303,103	$334,173	$366,139	$386,349
Leasehold					
improvements	$18,353	$18,353	$19,934	$19,934	$19,934
	$2,490,973	$2,512,539	$2,574,012	$2,630,029	$2,773,771
Less accumulated					
depreciation	$764,528	$891,650	$1,016,822	$1,144,886	$1,268,630
	$1,726,445	$1,620,889	$1,557,190	$1,485,143	$1,505,141
Total assets	$2,136,567	$2,148,203	$2,107,414	$2,141,374	$1,818,859
Current Liabilities					
Lease purchase					
agreement	$0	$0	$0	$0	$0
Bank overdraft	$19,998	$0	$0	$4,167	$0
Current maturities of					
long-term debt	$99,031	$179,235	$265,622	$294,528	$0
Accounts payable	$65,150	$68,712	$56,869	$73,279	$139,481
Accrued payroll	$20,673	$27,300	$35,055	$44,073	$51,509
Accrued lease payment	$0	$0	$0	$0	$0
Accrued interest	$56,679	$114,480	$32,232	$7,599	$6,696
Other accrued expenses	$31,331	$33,990	$38,987	$44,161	$41,861
Deferred revenue—					
Medicaid voluntary					
contributions	$0	$0	$0	$87,710	$0
Total current liabilities	$292,862	$423,717	$428,765	$555,517	$239,547
Long-term debt	$938,319	$856,874	$770,487	$678,975	$769,993
Fund balance	$905,386	$867,612	$908,162	$906,882	$809,319
Total liabilities and funds	$2,136,567	$2,148,203	$2,107,414	$2,141,374	$1,818,859

Table 1.3 Community Care Center Schedules of Operating Expenses Last Five Years

	5 Years Ago	4 Years Ago	3 Years Ago	2 Years Ago	Last Year
Nursing Services					
Salaries	$787,156	$927,446	$1,038,185	$1,172,006	$1,359,720
Professional fees	$18,738	$19,028	$21,918	$21,429	$17,643
Medical supplies	$61,438	$66,061	$62,214	$66,747	$128,027
	$867,332	$1,012,535	$1,122,317	$1,260,182	$1,505,390
Other (Pharmacy)					
Dietary					
Salaries	$142,036	$166,990	$181,586	$217,078	$297,706
Consultant	$0	$0	$0	$0	$0
Food cost	$184,779	$180,857	$185,302	$207,315	$205,508
Supplies	$23,418	$26,910	$26,386	$32,100	$33,241
	$350,233	$374,757	$393,274	$456,493	$536,455
Laundry					
Salaries	$36,239	$47,855	$57,008	$60,715	$56,474
Supplies	$22,832	$15,986	$22,309	$28,204	$24,938
	$59,071	$63,841	$79,317	$88,919	$81,412
Housekeeping					
Salaries	$115,465	$145,538	$167,631	$192,678	$204,925
Supplies	$28,976	$17,650	$20,609	$19,100	$16,691
	$144,441	$163,188	$188,240	$211,778	$221,616
Plant operations					
Salaries	$40,496	$48,445	$52,240	$55,383	$60,947
Rent	$867	$911	$976	$1,097	$1,372
Utilities	$109,407	$91,692	$96,565	$109,034	$92,258
Depreciation	$128,613	$127,122	$125,172	$128,064	$134,271
Supplies	$48,576	$46,052	$40,656	$44,579	$46,835
Maintenance	$11,974	$9,612	$38,409	$37,106	$34,436
	$339,933	$323,834	$354,018	$375,263	$370,119
General and administrative					
Salaries	$101,471	$138,692	$156,431	$133,067	$176,209
Payroll taxes	$91,776	$0	$0	$0	$0
Employee benefits	$88,094	$0	$0	$0	$0
Insurance	$64,715	$11,299	$8,182	$8,910	$9,816
Professional fees	$19,222	$21,771	$12,279	$11,291	$8,963
Bad debts	$22,541	$6,448	$16,926	$11,289	$8,996
Telephone	$4,164	$4,426	$4,336	$5,307	$6,040
Data processing	$259	$999	$5,519	$4,337	$1,167
Office supplies	$9,232	$10,926	$8,530	$8,312	$11,140
Interest	$62,799	$57,842	$53,096	$48,105	$42,930
Advertising	$976	$2,004	$5,336	$3,703	$2,570

Continued

Table 1.3 Continued

	5 Years Ago	4 Years Ago	3 Years Ago	2 Years Ago	Last Year
Vending machine supply	$18,266	$20,111	$16,457	$16,971	$8,815
Office equipment rental	$636	$2,506	$10,287	$0	$0
Training	$0	$0	$0	$5,574	$9,781
Loss on sale of fixed assets	$0	$0	$0	$0	$0
Miscellaneous	$6,464	$8,374	$7,596	$11,049	$17,369
	$490,615	$285,398	$304,975	$267,915	$303,796
	$2,251,625	$2,223,553	$2,442,141	$2,660,550	$3,018,788
Patient days					
Medicaid	28,928	27,407	29,320	29,264	30,233
Private and other	14,229	14,336	13,429	13,582	10,611
	43,157	41,743	42,749	42,846	40,844
Occupancy percent	96.7%	93.7%	96.0%	96.2%	91.7%
Medicaid % of occup.	67.0%	65.7%	68.6%	68.3%	74.0%
Per patient day					
Operating revenue	$49.76	$51.98	$55.23	$61.54	$63.90
Operating expense	$52.17	$53.27	$57.13	$62.80	$73.91
Operating revenue over operating expense	($2.41)	($1.29)	($1.90)	($1.26)	($10.01)

Problems Begin to Surface

After 1987, the facility began experiencing more persistent problems. Food problems resisted solution, and there was a fairly pervasive negative attitude on the part of a small, but vocal, group of residents' families about the poor food and the administrator's lack of concern for residents. Additionally, the facility increasingly began to experience problems with state inspections. While cited deficiencies were often corrected in a short-term way, the same problems repeatedly were documented.

Four years ago, a new county commissioner was elected and joined the CCC board. He disliked the current administrator and frequently attacked his leadership, problem solving, and financial management performance. He also expressed a concern that the board needed to assume policy control of the facility. The commissioner's style incurred the resentment of several board members, especially from the ranks of long-term members who felt he was trying to change the rules in the middle of the game, and that his attacks were divisive and overly critical.

Table 1.4 Staffing: Full-Time Equivalents

	Norms*	Pay† Period 1	Pay Period 2	Pay Period 3	Pay Period 4	Pay Period 5	10 Week Average
Accounting	2.1	3.00	3.00	3.00	3.01	3.06	3.014
Nursing							
RN	2.6	4.12	3.95	4.00	3.56	4.02	3.930
LPN	8.4	12.92	14.32	15.06	16.07	12.35	14.144
Aides	48.5	51.81	50.40	50.53	51.24	47.02	50.200
Social service	1.1	1.70	1.00	1.02	1.22	1.25	1.238
Dietary	14.2	22.53	18.31	19.90	18.14	17.00	19.176
Laundry	6.2	3.35	2.89	3.25	3.58	3.57	3.328
Houskeeping	9.7	15.08	13.85	12.27	13.82	13.23	13.650
Maintenance	3.1	2.00	2.00	2.00	2.00	2.00	2.000
Administration	4.2	5.62	4.93	5.61	5.63	5.70	5.498

*Norms suggested by firm auditing CCC and other nursing facilities.
†Five pay periods prior to consultants' arrival.

During this period the management firm that ran the county hospital approached the county commission about possibly also managing the nursing home. For political reasons, the commissioner did not want to seriously entertain this notion, but he felt that it afforded him leverage to force the board to address facility problems.

In an effort to delay further consideration of the contract management proposition and to bring to the surface the problems plaguing CCC, the commissioner and several allies on the board urged the full board to engage an outside consultant to develop a strategic plan. To make it more palatable for reluctant board members, the commissioner agreed that the county would fund the strategic planning study. A request for proposals was solicited from several organizations, and a private consulting firm was selected to assist with strategic planning.

II: Crises Erupt

CCC Makes the Press

In the midst of considering strategic planning, a reporter for a local radio station began an investigative report that resulted in an extremely critical news story broadcast during two lengthy evening reports. The following day the story was picked up by the two local newspapers in front page stories. The charges, drawn from interviews with disgruntled former employees and several residents' family members, included bad food, poor care, poor staff relations, extremely high staff turnover, and general assertions that the facility was poorly managed and the board was neglecting its oversight responsibility. The reporter reviewed the state surveys of the last seven years and found that they chronicled a range of issues that substantiated these allegations.

CCC's Response

The administrator's response to this negative publicity was to stonewall the press and any others who sought information about the charges. The board, caught off guard by the stories, at first was disorganized in its response. Several members refused to talk to the press. Two others stated that it appeared the administrator was not doing his job, a statement that appeared in a follow-up newspaper article. The county commissioner, anxious about the political ramifications, quietly urged the board to request an evaluation by an independent citizen's group. When the results of the past state surveys became known through the news articles, the board acknowledged it had never seen them before. The administrator stated it had not been his practice to "go into details" with the board.

The board met quickly, in closed session, with Mr. Dolinsky. It requested a copy of the most recent survey and reviewed its findings. Mr. Dolinsky felt the problems cited were being addressed, and that the deficiencies were not widespread or enduring, but the result of recent staffing problems. The board demanded Dolinsky immediately develop a plan of correction as required by the state. Next, it passed a resolution requesting that the county commission appoint a citizen's board of inquiry to independently audit the care being provided.

Mr. Dolinsky prepared a plan of correction, which the state rejected as not specifically addressing the deficiencies. Later, at its October meeting, the board reviewed Dolinsky's plan. The 60-page survey document was very specific. Dolinsky's 20-page response challenged some of its findings, was vague about compliance, and generally lacked much substance.

The commissioner became outraged, and charged Mr. Dolinsky with jeopardizing the future of the facility and not addressing the seriousness of the situation. Dolinsky reacted defensively, stating he felt the state's review was unfair, unreasonable, and provided no guidelines for him to follow. The board, however, pushed Dolinsky to be more specific. Dolinsky's revised plan was accepted by the state later that month.

The Citizen's Committee Review

In November, the citizen's committee conducted its on-site review of the facility, and presented its report in early December. During the assessment volunteers, employees, and several residents and their families were interviewed. Committee members came away with a sense of a facility that was drifting, lacking leadership and management. Their report substantiated the deficiencies cited by the state. They criticized the director of nursing's lack of supervisory skills and failure to take sufficient action to remedy care problems. The committee also criticized Dolinsky's neglect of care issues and the absence of executive leadership; it furthermore chastised the board for its failure to provide sufficient monitoring and oversight. The committee was additionally concerned that negative press coverage had damaged the morale of the staff to the point where long-time, formerly loyal employees were talking of leaving.

The Board's Response

Several board members, led by the county commissioner, were upset at Dolinsky's flagrant failure to inform them about CCC's affairs, and mounted an attempt to fire him. This culminated in a closed board meeting in which there was a heated debate about the problems and how to deal with them. The board was divided on what to do about the administrator. All were concerned about his performance. Three members thought Mr. Dolinsky should be summarily terminated. Some board members believed, since they had not clearly laid out their expectations beforehand, that it would be unfair to fire him without giving him some opportunity to change. The older board members were in a quandary since, to them, it did not appear that Dolinsky was performing any differently than he had for the last twenty years when his management of the facility had been considered acceptable. Most board members simply thought it would be too difficult to replace him while the facility was under public scrutiny and attack.

The board finally agreed to place Dolinsky on probation and require him to develop a plan of action to address the citizen's committee report. Mr. Dolinsky was informed of its decision and requested to present his plan the following month.

Shortly thereafter, Ms. Babcock, the director of nursing, suddenly announced her retirement. Mr. Dolinsky, unable to recruit a replacement, persuaded a veteran floor nurse, Sandy Long, to assume the position. Ms. Long lacked supervisory experience, but agreed to take the position on an interim basis. The next month the state review team returned for a follow-up inspection. It was apparently satisfied with the progress being made.

The negative publicity had, however, taken its toll. Several private pay residents moved to other facilities and admissions dropped off precipitously. Occupancy fell from an average of 91 percent to 83 percent, and remained at that level for the rest of the year. This exacerbated the already shaky financial situation of the organization.

The board did not know how to proceed. It met to review the administrator's work plan and found it limited in scope and lacking insight into the real problems of the organization. The meeting turned into a brainstorming session in which various members attempted to develop ideas for improving the situation. At this point, the board also decided it should seek outside assistance immediately, in order to address its pressing concerns.

III: Consultation and Actions

The board and administrator met with the consultants seeking advice on how to proceed and to help define their respective roles and responsibilities. The consultants recommended damage control, including addressing all serious internal problems, before developing a strategic plan.

After a brief review of materials, interviews with board members, the administrator, key staff, and an assessment of CCC's operational structure, the consultants presented the board with three recommendations:

1. Redefine the administrator's job description to strengthen the board's executive management expectations and plan a performance evaluation to be conducted six months after the initial probation by the board
2. Strengthen CCC's basic policies and operational structure, especially in human resources
3. Institute a development session to strengthen the board's understanding of its roles and responsibilities.

The board agreed to implement the consultants' recommendations and requested their help in monitoring the administrator's performance. During the next several months, the consultants worked with the administrator in revising job descriptions and designing and delivering board training sessions. The board was quite receptive to these sessions. As a result, the members began reviewing financial reports carefully and requested that the administrator present monthly information about admissions, discharges, problems in the facility, and employee turnover.

The county commissioner was becoming discouraged and alarmed. He was convinced that neither the board nor the administrator were moving fast enough to turn things around or reverse the considerable loss which had resulted from decreasing occupancy. In addition, CCC was continuously in arrears on its lease payments. The commissioner's main concern, however, was the negative public reaction which was sure to ensue if CCC were to become financially insolvent. He believed both he and the commission would be roundly criticized for not fulfilling their fiduciary obligations. Furthermore, the care and well-being of the county's citizens would be jeopardized.

The consultants found working with the administrator to be quite challenging. Mr. Dolinsky readily accepted the ideas presented by the consulting group, but seemed to have none of his own. Ideas and plans he did put forth seemed ill-conceived, and their implications not well thought out. Mr. Dolinsky was not up to the job; thus the consultants were in a quandary. If they were more forceful in promoting their ideas, potential successes might further mask the administrator's shortcomings and make it more difficult for the board to assess his performance. On the other hand, it was increasingly evident that the administrator was not providing the kind of leadership and management the facility needed.

The six months' probationary period passed and the time for Mr. Dolinsky's performance review approached. The board asked the consultants to assist in the process. The board had, with the consultant's assistance, developed a comprehensive job description, and the functions it described were the basis for their assessment. The consultants met with the executive committee to develop the evaluation document. It was then completed by board members and analyzed by the consultants prior to discussion with the administrator.

The results were quite equivocal. Several board members wrote that they believed the administrator probably should be terminated. The administrator's overall evaluation was that his performance was "adequate." Analysis of individual responses indicated that more than half of the board members felt that Dolinsky was performing below average in most areas. In fact, if the evaluations of three long-term board members, who rated the performance better than average in several categories, were not included, the overall average was much lower.

At the board meeting there was protracted discussion of both the basis for the performance evaluation and the evaluation itself. There was general agreement that Dolinsky's performance was below expectations, but far from agreement on what action to take. Several members were still reluctant to terminate an administrator they had worked with for 20 years.

One board member finally introduced a motion to terminate Mr. Dolinsky. It was seconded by the commissioner. With eight of the nine board members present, the vote was four to three against the motion, with one abstention. In exasperation, the board voted to extend the administrator's probationary period for another six months. If his performance did not improve by the end of the year, then he would be terminated.

Over the next three months, the facility's financial condition deteriorated, with little improvement in admissions and occupancy levels. One board member who originally voted against firing Mr. Dolinsky contacted the consultants and indicated she now felt he should be terminated. The consultants suggested she contact other board members and share her views and concerns. If there seemed to be a majority with that opinion, a group of three board members could go to Dolinsky and ask him to resign. She followed the consultants' advice, and to her amazement, when the group went to the administrator, he readily agreed to resign.

This accomplished, the board appointed the assistant administrator to an acting capacity and engaged the consultants to assist in recruiting and hiring a new administrator. Shortly thereafter, the state surveyors again came in for CCC's annual inspection.

The Survey Report

The facility was cited by the state as providing substandard care, based on the outcome of a week-long inspection. Three Level A deficiencies, the most serious type, were recorded in the areas of quality of life, quality of care, and administration. The 93-page list of findings and deficiencies also included numerous Level B deficiencies in areas ranging from sanitation to the delivery of patient care. The findings were even more serious when considered in light of the past two annual state inspections, both of which cited Level A deficiencies in the same areas. As a result, new admissions were banned for 60 days and nurse aide training could not be conducted by the facility for 24 months.

The year-end audit indicated a net loss of over $400,000. This was the fifth consecutive year that the facility had reported a net loss; by the end of May losses were approximately $21,000 per month. The financial crisis became so acute, the facility no longer had cash available to meet biweekly payrolls. The state further ordered the facility to provide an immediate plan to demonstrate financial viability.

During May the facility was notified that worker's compensation coverage would be canceled by the state Nursing Home Insurance Trust as a result of the substandard nature of operations. The property, liability, and casualty insurers of the facility also notified officials of the termination of coverage effective July 1, as a result of state survey findings and the impending financial crisis.

The facility had no current policies or procedures manual; department heads were operating with relative independence in the conduct of their respective departments. The activities department had the highest costs of any in the state, while the food service department had an average daily meal cost more than double the state norm. CCC was the only facility in the area with a full-time registered dietician providing a menu selection for residents. Residents made choices from up to fifteen offerings, even though half of the residents were cognitively impaired.

Needless to say, the acting administrator, and then his permanent replacement, and the board had their work cut out for them. The pressing question was where to begin.

Ridgecrest Nursing Facility: Information Technology Facilitating Quality Improvement

William T. Reddick and Diane K. Duin

BUILDING ON past and current initiatives for quality assurance and an equitable Medicare and Medicaid payment system, the Health Care Financing Administration (HCFA) in 1989 funded the Nursing Home Case Mix and Quality demonstration. Four states—Kansas, Maine, Mississippi, and South Dakota—entered into cooperative agreements with HCFA to initiate demonstrations that would promote Title XIX objectives. The purpose of the demonstration was to test a resident information system with variables for care planning; classifying residents into homogeneous resource utilization groups; and monitoring process and outcomes, adjusted for case mix. The original HFCA minimum data set (MDS) was intended as a resident data collection tool whose functionality was embellished through several modifications: (1) additional items for resident classification by resource utilization, (2) additional items for the payment system, (3) items required for quality assurance monitoring, and (4) items essential for a research and evaluation database. Because of the revised functionality of the MDS system for both quality monitoring and payment classification, as well as extra process variables for foot care, rehabilitation, and nursing procedures to assist in matching process to outcomes, the new moniker was given, MDS+ (see Appendix 2.1).

This case is based on a composite of experiences in three South Dakota nursing homes. The names of the facility and the people involved have been fictionalized to permit the utilization of certain facts.

Figure 2.1 Ridgecrest Nursing Facility Organization Chart

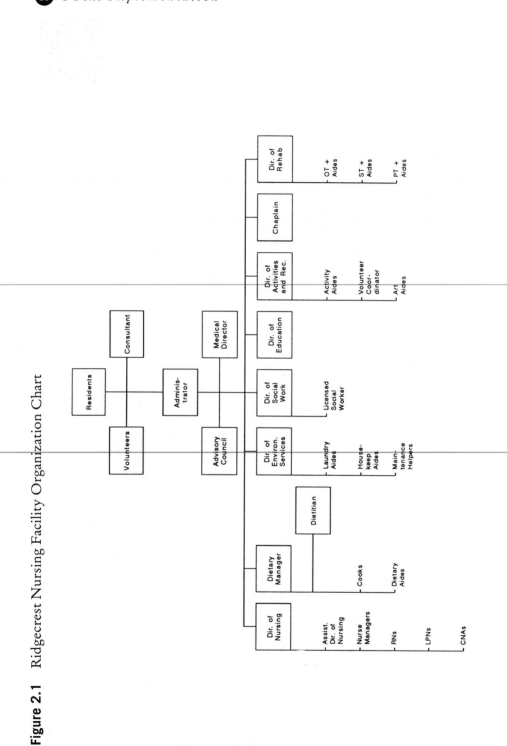

The State Perspective

As the administrative agent, the state became responsible for oversight, compliance, and certification to HCFA that its nursing facilities had either met the requirements of the new standards or were in the process of a time-phased plan of correction to remedy any deficiency. If a facility had not met the requirements, the state was also responsible for resurveying it within 90 days to assess and reevaluate compliance.

The implementation of the federally legislated mandate in South Dakota represents a five-year process of design, planning, experimentation, initiation of state legislation, staff training, facility training, analysis, and refinement. Because of its participation in the Nursing Home Case Mix and Quality Demonstration, South Dakota essentially pioneered real-time case-mix micromanagement using the MDS+ system. According to the Office of Program Management—Adult Services and Aging, South Dakota is the only state with a resident-specific, computerized case-mix system. Entering a parallel transition stage (manual and computerized records both transmitted for reimbursement) at the end of July, South Dakota began statewide microcomputer-based reporting using software conforming to the MDS+ database specifications. Although a manual system was begun in the fall following the OBRA '87 mandate, the system has been fully automated as of this January. Utilizing intensive training, proactive management, computerized review, and appropriate intervention, South Dakota has successfully and effectively implemented the MDS+ system for reimbursement in the care of its approximately 4,500 Medicaid nursing home residents.

The Nursing Facility Perspective

Kay Thompson has been the administrator at the Ridgecrest Nursing Facility for five years. (see Figure 2.1 for organization chart.) Ridgecrest, located in Siouxland, South Dakota, is a 65-bed, stand-alone nursing facility situated in a rural community with a population of about 18,000. The Ridgecrest case mix is 60 percent Medicaid and 40 percent private pay. Ridgecrest is not licensed for Medicare beds. The other local nursing facility, Siouxgate Municipal Nursing Facility, has 90 beds and is attached to Siouxgate Municipal Hospital. The Siouxgate Municipal Nursing Facility is licensed for five Medicare beds. The typical patient mix for Siouxgate Municipal Nursing Facility includes 52 private pay, 36 Medicaid, and 2 Medicare patients.

South Dakota Implements Medicaid Case-Mix Management

Ms. Thompson had read and attended meetings over the last two years regarding the implementation of the new South Dakota case-mix management software, MDS+. She felt challenged by all of the changes she believed this new system of Medicaid reimbursement required of her facility. At the same time, she believed the eventual benefits to patient care in the facility will outweigh any problems she recently had been encountering.

The first major challenge Ms. Thompson faced with the implementation of MDS+ was the purchase of a computer system for Ridgecrest Nursing Facility. Ridgecrest did not use a computer system at all until two years ago. Ms. Thompson worked with the bookkeeper to decide on a system and a vendor for the software that was required for the MDS+ system. The bookkeeper, Jean South, indicated that she was willing to learn the computer system and to input data on the required forms. Ms. Thompson later learned, however, that OBRA '87 regulations permit only an RN or LPN to input data on the MDS+ form.

Ridgecrest Responds to the MDS+ System

Last year, Ms. Thompson decided to have Linda Ryan, an LPN who had been working part-time nights, trained in computer use and eventually work with the MDS+ system. Following routine procedures, Ms. Thompson had requested a personnel posting for the position.

When she had read the formal announcement for an RN or LPN to function as the part-time MDS Coordinator, Linda Ryan quickly applied for the position. Linda was anxious to learn all about MDS+ and to work with Ms. Thompson in implementing the system. Initially, Linda continued to work two nights a week on the floor, as well as two days during the week learning the MDS+ system. She attended several workshops at the State Department of Social Services during the implementation phase. The six months prior to full implementation of MDS+ was a very busy period. Linda found herself spending more and more of her days off at the facility working on the MDS+ system. One month prior to full implementation, Ms. Thompson asked Linda if she would consider working as the full-time MDS Coordinator. Because she has two young children and enjoyed being home in the afternoons when they returned from school, Linda was reluctant. But since she had been spending so much time working with the system, she decided to take the full-time position, thinking that her time would at least be structured and she would be able to get home when she needed to.

Now Linda is finding that she must frequently return to the facility in the evenings and on weekends to complete data input, especially since she shares the computer with Jean South, the bookkeeper. Linda is considering approaching Ms. Thompson to request that another person be hired and trained to assist her. If not, Linda is considering resigning. She thinks she will be able to work for the Siouxgate Municipal Nursing Facility. After all, yesterday she saw an advertisement in the local paper for a part-time LPN.

The MDS+ System Alters Resource Requirements

Ms. Thompson recently realized that another computer might have to be purchased for Jean South. The facility billing system had been placed on computer about eighteen months ago. Jean has been complaining that it is difficult to get the bookkeeping completed with Linda needing to use the computer so much for MDS+ data input. Jean also is frustrated with Linda hovering around, constantly asking when she will be finished using the computer. Linda told Jean she was coming in during the evening hours and on the weekends to get her work done, and she had made it sound like it was Jean's fault she had to take the time away from her family. Jean has had to utilize the computer system to generate an MDS+ assessment on every resident in order to accurately determine the case mix of the facility and justify the base level of payment. Ms. Thompson has noticed the growing conflict between Jean and Linda over computer access. She is concerned about the cost of another computer and feels frustrated at the overall cost to the facility resulting from implementation of the MDS+ system. She hopes that increases in revenue from Medicaid due to the new levels of reimbursement will be enough, over time, to offset the additional capital costs.

MDS+ Demands Timely Reporting

Linda Ryan has carefully coordinated the care conferences for each resident. Care conferences and the MDS+ have to be completed within seven days of the assessment. During the implementation phase, when a parallel paper filing to the state was used, along with the electronic filing for the MDS+ system, several of the MDS+ assessments were returned because a crosscheck revealed the reporting date to not be within seven days of the actual assessment. This occurred only a few times in the early implementation of the electronic system, and resulted in delay of payment to the facility. Although the fully implemented system has checks against such a recurrence, Linda quickly adapted an elaborate and accurate schedule for assuring that resident care conferences are completed on time, immediately followed by the completion of the MDS+. She has now incorporated due dates for resident reassessments into her schedule. She makes certain that Ms. Thompson, as well as every department head in the facility, has a copy of the schedule. Linda has not learned a way to work with this schedule on the computer, so currently she is working it out by hand each week. She has discovered there are some problems between what she and the state determine as the due date for the reassessment. Linda asked Ms. Thompson how to handle such discrepancies, and they decided to use what the state reports, since it is that type of error which results in delays of payment to the facility.

Conflict and Resolution

Linda is frustrated with the way the state is handling problems with the MDS+ data and has frequently shared her frustration with Ms. Thompson. It doesn't matter if it is her error or the state's, she always is responsible for correcting the problem. This frequently results in a delay in the reimbursement, which Linda feels makes her "look bad."

Facility Coordination

The MDS+ system required changes in the involvement of department heads in care conferences. Prior to implementation Ms. Thompson included discussions on these changes at weekly department head meetings. She talked about how important it would be for those in dietary, physical therapy, activities, and social work to provide equal input at the care conference. Since the MDS+ system uses each data element in measuring the amount of care given to each resident, she stressed the importance of noting specifically what is done for each resident. She expressed her concern to department heads that this was a significant change from the way things were done before, when only nursing service created care plans, and others went along with what needed to be done. Ms. Thompson believes department heads are contributing to care coordination and she continues to discuss the topic at department head meetings in order to bring any concerns to the surface before they become major problems.

Quality Care Tied to Reimbursement Levels

Alice Kessler, director of nursing, has been meeting with Ms. Thompson on a regular basis to discuss how MDS+ implementation is affecting the nursing service. Alice has recently discussed some significant changes in staffing. Use of the MDS+ system made her aware that labor-intensive facilities are rewarded. She has been carefully studying and discussing the MDS+ with Linda, and both of them realize that the more that is done for the residents, the better the quality of care will be and, subsequently, the higher the level of reimbursement.

Increasing the FTE of Nursing Aides

Recently, Alice began to reevaluate the impact of nursing aides on the care given to residents. She conducted time studies with the nursing aides and determined that the number of times the aides have the residents up and walking during the day and the number of activities the residents are involved in affects the reimbursement level. Working with Linda on the MDS+ data, Alice has learned that it will be more beneficial to residents if nursing aides put out meal trays. Also, she wants nursing aides to pass out afternoon and evening snacks. This traditionally has been the duty of dietary aides, but Alice is certain the dietary supervisor will not be disturbed if the nursing aides assume some of the dietary aides' duties. It shouldn't make too much difference in the number of work hours available to the dietary aides. However, all of these extra duties have put something of a strain on the nursing aides.

Alice has routinely utilized five nursing aides each day and on evening shifts, with three nursing aides on night shifts. Recently, she talked with Ms. Thompson about increasing the number of nursing aides on the day shift. Alice believes she can justify the increase based on the increase in nursing aide duties and the amount of time each aide is spending with each resident. She believes that if there is another aide available to increase the ratio of aides to residents, she can change the level of care to increase the reimbursement on the Medicaid residents. Her problem at this time is that she must consider what impact this will have on private pay residents, since she cannot discriminate. She realizes she will not be able to increase private pay rates, and that aides will have to provide the same amount of care to them as to Medicaid residents. Her discussions with Ms. Thompson have focused on whether there will be enough of an increase in Medicaid reimbursement to offset the cost of the new nursing aide without increasing the cost to private pay residents. Ms. Thompson is "working on the numbers" prior to making a decision.

Working with Outside Consultants

Ron Robbins is the consultant physical therapist who works at Ridgecrest three days per week. Ron has one physical therapy aide, who handles the necessary duties on the two days per week Ron is not there and works with Ron one day a week. Ron tries to involve himself as much as possible in residents' care conferences, but he also consults at a nursing facility in a neighboring town and finds he cannot always be at Ridgecrest when the care conferences are scheduled. Ron has complete confidence in Marybeth Barnes, his physical therapy aide. Marybeth has been working with Ron for the past seven years at Ridgecrest, and probably knows more than Ron about each resident. He has asked Marybeth to sit in on the care conferences when he is not available.

Yesterday, Alice Kessler talked with Ron about hiring an additional physical therapy aide to be available on the weekends and to provide more restorative care to the residents. Ron is aware of the new MDS+ system, but he is not quite sure how it all works. He really hasn't had time to attend many department head meetings. Actually, Ron thinks Kay Thompson holds too many department head meetings. If she would organize the meetings better and not waste so much time, she could accomplish as much in a meeting held every other week, instead of requiring a weekly meeting. The administrator before Ms. Thompson held monthly department head meetings, and Ron was able to attend most of those.

Alice talked to Ron about increasing the level of reimbursement from Medicaid by doing more restorative care, such as walking and rotating limbs, on each of the residents. She would like Ron to consider hiring additional staff. Ron is not sure how increasing his staff will increase revenue. He is concerned that by hiring another physical therapy aide his net revenue will decrease, and he just doesn't want to deal with Ms. Thompson's reaction to that. Besides, Ron believes that he and Marybeth are doing just fine with the residents' physical therapy. Ron told Alice he would think about it and get back to her later. As far as he is concerned, it will be much later.

Is the Information System Facilitating Quality of Care?

Kay Thompson was aware when she purchased the MDS+ software program that it contained a quality indicator portion, but neither Jean nor Linda have learned how to use that portion of the software yet. She recently has been reading the information the vendor provided regarding data she can generate from the MDS+ concerning quality indicators. Ms. Thompson is aware that the state is generating quality indicators from the data submitted to them, but at this point they are not using it for any purpose. Last Saturday, when Ms. Thompson was in the office, she sat down at the computer and tried to generate quality indicators from the MDS+. Today, she has been comparing the data generated from the computer with the data she has from the quality assurance committee; they do not look similar. Ms. Thompson is concerned that the state soon will want to use the quality indicators in their surveys. She is afraid that it

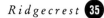

may indicate a problem, and would like to know prior to any survey what problems might exist at Ridgecrest. Ms. Thompson thinks she should have a talk with Linda next week about learning the quality indicator portion of the computer program and getting it up and going in the very near future. Perhaps she could set that as a goal for Linda next month.

Appendix 2.1

DSS - AA - 655 - 12/1/90B

STATE OF SOUTH DAKOTA
MINIMUM DATA SET PLUS FOR NURSING HOME RESIDENT ASSESSMENT AND CARE SCREENING (MDS+)

Part I

BACKGROUND INFORMATION AT INTAKE/ADMISSION

I. IDENTIFICATION INFORMATION

1.	RESIDENT NAME	First: _____ Last: _____		M.I. _____	
2.	DATE OF CURRENT ADMISSION	Month — Day — Year			
3.	MEDICARE NO. (SOC. SEC. or Comparable No. if no Medicare No.)				
4.	FACILITY PROVIDER NO.	Federal No.			
5.	GENDER	1. Male 2. Female			
6.	RACE/ ETHNICITY	1. American Indian/Alaska Native 4. Hispanic 2. Asian/Pacific Islander 5. White, not of Hispanic origin 3. Black, not of Hispanic origin			
7.	BIRTHDATE	Month — Day — Year			
8.	LIFETIME OCCUPA- TION				
9.	PRIMARY LANGUAGE	Resident's primary language is language other than English. 0. No 1. Yes _____ (Specify)			

II. BACKGROUND INFORMATION AT RETURN/READMISSION

1.	DATE OF CURRENT READMIS- SION	Month — Day — Year
2.	MARITAL STATUS	1. Never Married 3. Widowed 5. Divorced 2. Married 4. Separated
3.	ADMITTED FROM	1. Private home or apt. 3. Acute care hospital 2. Nursing home 4. Other
4.	LIVED ALONE	0. No 1. Yes 2. In other facility

III. CUSTOMARY ROUTINE (ONLY AT FIRST ADMISSION)

CUSTOMARY ROUTINE (Year prior to first admission to a nursing home)	(Check all that apply. If all information is UNKNOWN, check last box only.)	
	1. CYCLE OF DAILY EVENTS	
	Stays up late at night (e.g., after 9 pm)	a.
	Naps regularly during day (at least 1 hour)	b.
	Goes out 1+ days a week	c.
	Stays busy with hobbies, reading, or fixed daily routine	d.
	Spends most time alone or watching TV	e.
	Moves independently indoors (with appliances, if used)	f.
	Use of tobacco products at least daily	g.
	NONE OF ABOVE	h.
	2. EATING PATTERNS	

10.	RESIDENTIAL HISTORY PAST 5 YEARS	(Check all settings resident lived in during 5 years prior to admission)	
		Prior stay at this nursing home	a.
		Other nursing home/residential facility	b.
		MH/psychiatric setting	c.
		MR/DD setting	d.
		NONE OF ABOVE	e.
11.	MENTAL HEALTH HISTORY	Does resident's RECORD indicate any history of mental retardation, mental illness, or any other mental health problem?　0. No　1. Yes	
12.	CONDITIONS RELATED TO MR/DD STATUS	Check all conditions that are related to MR/DD Status, that were manifested before age 22, and are likely to continue indefinitely.	
		Not applicable - no MR/DD (Skip to Item 13)	a.
		MR/DD with Organic Condition	
		Cerebral palsy	b.
		Down's syndrome	c.
		Autism	d.
		Epilepsy	e.
		Other organic condition related to MR/DD	f.
		MR/DD with no organic condition	g.
		Unknown	h.
13.	MARITAL STATUS	1. Never married　3. Widowed　5. Divorced 2. Married　4. Separated	
14.	ADMITTED FROM	1. Private home or apt.　3. Acute care hospital 2. Nursing home　4. Other	
15.	LIVED ALONE	0. No　1. Yes　2. In other facility	
16.	ADMISSION INFORMATION AMENDED	(Check all that apply)	
		Accurate information unavailable earlier	a.
		Observation revealed additional information	b.
		Resident unstable at admission	c.

Distinct food preferences		i.
Eats between meals all or most days		j.
Use of alcoholic beverages(s) at least weekly		k.
NONE OF ABOVE		l.
3. ADL PATTERNS		
In bed/clothes much of day		m.
Wakens to toilet all or most nights		n.
Has irregular bowel movement pattern		o.
Prefers showers for bathing		p.
Prefers bathing in P.M.		q.
NONE OF ABOVE		r.
4. INVOLVEMENT PATTERNS		
Daily contact with relatives/close friends		s.
Usually attends church, temple, synagogue (etc.)		t.
Finds strength in faith		u.
Daily animal companion/presence		v.
Involved in group activities		w.
NONE OF ABOVE		x.
UNKNOWN - Resident/family unable to provide information		y.

MEDICAL RECORD NO.

DOCUMENT NO.

CORRECTION DOCUMENT NO.

License Number

Signature of RN Assessment Coordinator: _____

Signatures of Others Who Completed Part of the Assessment: _____

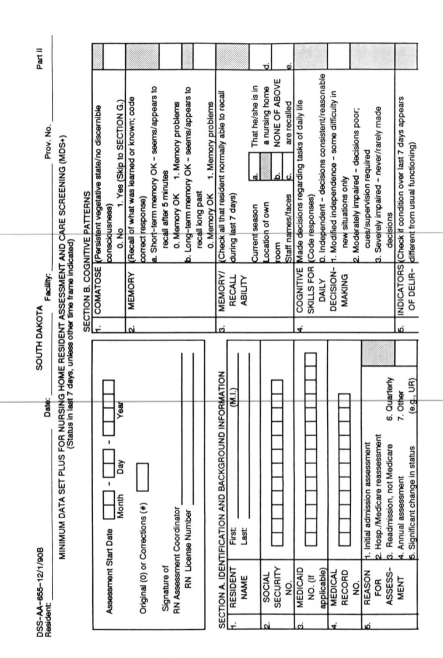

DSS-AA-655-12/1/90B   Date: _____   SOUTH DAKOTA   Facility: _____   Prov. No. _____   Part II

Resident: _____

MINIMUM DATA SET PLUS FOR NURSING HOME RESIDENT ASSESSMENT AND CARE SCREENING (MDS+)

(Status in last 7 days, unless other time frame indicated)

Assessment Start Date ☐☐ - ☐☐ - ☐☐
Month Day Year

Original (0) or Corrections (#) ☐

Signature of
RN Assessment Coordinator _____
RN License Number _____

SECTION A. IDENTIFICATION AND BACKGROUND INFORMATION

1.	RESIDENT NAME	First: _____ Last: _____	(M.I.)	
2.	SOCIAL SECURITY NO.			☐☐☐☐☐
3.	MEDICAID NO. (If applicable)			☐☐☐☐☐
4.	MEDICAL RECORD NO.			☐☐☐☐☐
5.	REASON FOR ASSESS-MENT	1. Initial admission assessment 2. Hosp./Medicare reassessment 6. Quarterly 3. Readmission, not Medicare 7. Other 4. Annual assessment 5. Significant change in status (e.g., UR)		☐

SECTION B. COGNITIVE PATTERNS

1.	COMATOSE	(Persistent vegetative state/no discernible consciousness) 0. No 1. Yes (Skip to SECTION G.)	☐

2.	MEMORY	(Recall of what was learned or known; code correct response)
		a. Short-term memory OK – seems/appears to recall after 5 minutes
		   0. Memory OK 1. Memory problems
		b. Long-term memory OK – seems/appears to recall long past
		   0. Memory OK 1. Memory problems
			☐
			
			☐

3.	MEMORY/ RECALL ABILITY	(Check all that resident normally able to recall during last 7 days) Current season a. ☐ Location of own room That he/she is in a nursing home b. ☐ Staff names/faces NONE OF ABOVE are recalled c. ☐	
4.	COGNITIVE SKILLS FOR DAILY DECISION-MAKING	Made decisions regarding tasks of daily life (Code responses) 0. Independent – decisions consistent/reasonable 1. Modified independence – some difficulty in new situations only 2. Moderately impaired – decisions poor; cues/supervision required 3. Severely impaired – never/rarely made decisions	☐
5.	INDICATORS OF DELIR-	(Check if condition over last 7 days appears different from usual functioning)	d. ☐ e. ☐

6.	CURRENT PAYMENT SOURCE(S) FOR NH STAY	(Billing Office to code payment sources) 0. Not used 1. Per diem 2. Ancillary 3. Both	
		Medicaid [ ]	VA [ ]
		Medicare [ ]	Self pay/Private insur. [ ]
		CHAMPUS [ ]	Other [ ]

7.	RESPONSI-BILITY/ LEGAL GUARDIAN	(Check all that apply)		
		Legal guardian	Family member responsible	a. [ ]
		Other legal oversight	Resident responsible	b. [ ]
		Durable power attrny./ health care proxy	None of above	c. [ ] d. e. f.

8.	ADVANCED DIRECTIVES	(For those items with supporting documentation in the medical record, check all that apply)		
		Living will	a.	Feeding restrictions	f.
		Do not resuscitate	b.	Medication restric-tions	g.
		Do not hospitalize	c.	Other treatment restrictions	h.
		Organ donation	d.	NONE OF ABOVE	i.
		Autopsy request	e.		

9.	DISCHARGE PLANNED WITHIN 3 MOS.	(Does not include discharge due to death) 0. No 1. Yes 2. Unknown/uncertain

10.	MARITAL STATUS	1. Never married 4. Separated
		2. Married 5. Divorced
		3. Widowed

6.	- IUM /PERIODIC DIS-ORDERED THINKING/ AWARE-NESS	Less alert, easily distracted	a.
		Changing awareness of environment	b.
		Episodes of incoherent speech	c.
		Periods of motor restlessness or lethargy	d.
		Cognitive ability varies over course of day	e.
		NONE OF ABOVE	f.

6.	CHANGE IN COGNITIVE STATUS	Change in resident's cognitive status, skills, or abilities – in last 90 days	
		0. No change 1. Improved 2. Deteriorated	

SECTION C. COMMUNICATION/HEARING PATTERNS

1.	HEARING	(With hearing appliance, if used)	
		0. Hears adequately – normal talk, TV, phone	
		1. Minimal difficulty when not in quiet setting	
		2. Hears in special situation only – speaker has to adjust tonal quality and speak distinctly	
		3. Highly impaired/absence of useful hearing	

2.	COMMUNI-CATION DEVICES/ TECH-NIQUES	(Check all that apply during last 7 days)	
		Hearing aid, present and used	a.
		Hearing aid, present and not used	b.
		Other receptive comm. technique used (e.g., lip read)	c.
		NONE OF ABOVE	d.

Code the appropriate response = [ ]

Check all the responses that apply = [b.]

Resident: _____ Date: _____ Facility: _____ Prov. No. _____

MINIMUM DATA SET PLUS FOR NURSING HOME RESIDENT ASSESSMENT AND CARE SCREENING (MDS+)
(Status in last 7 days, unless other time frame indicated)

SECTION C. CONT.

3. MODES OF EXPRESSION (Check all used by resident to make needs known)

Speech	a.
Writing messages to express or clarify needs	b.
Signs/gestures/sounds	c.
Communication board	d.
American Sign Language or Braille	e.
Other	f.
NONE OF ABOVE	g.

4. MAKING SELF UNDERSTOOD (Expressing information content – however able)
0. Understood
1. Usually understood -- difficulty finding words or finishing thoughts
2. Sometimes understood -- ability is limited to making concrete requests
3. Rarely/never understood

5. SPEECH CLARITY Speech unclear
0. No   1. Yes

6. ABILITY TO UNDERSTAND OTHERS (Understanding verbal information content – however able)
0. Understands
1. Usually understands -- may miss some part/intent of message
2. Sometimes understands -- responds adequately to simple, direct communication
3. Rarely/never understands

7. CHANGE IN COMMUNICATION/HEARING Resident's ability to express, understand or hear information has changed over last 90 days
0. No change   1. Improved   2. Deteriorated

SECTION E. MOOD AND BEHAVIOR PATTERNS

1. SAD OR ANXIOUS MOOD (Check all that apply during last 30 days)

VERBAL EXPRESSIONS of DISTRESS by resident (sadness, sense that nothing matters, hopelessness, worthlessness, unrealistic fears, vocal expressions of anxiety or grief) — a.

DEMONSTRATED (OBSERVABLE) SIGNS of mental DISTRESS
- Tearfulness, emotional groaning, sighing, breathlessness — b.
- Motor agitation such as pacing, handwringing or picking — c.
- Pervasive concern with health — d.
- Recurrent thoughts of death – e.g., believes he/she about to die, have a heart attack — e.
- Suicidal thoughts/actions — f.
- Failure to eat or take medications — g.
- Withdrawal from self-care, or leisure activities — h.
- Reduced communications — i.
- Early morning awakening with unpleasant mood — j.
NONE OF ABOVE — k.

2. MOOD PERSISTENCE Sad or anxious mood intrudes on daily life over last 7 days – not easily altered, doesn't "cheer up"
0. No   1. Yes

3. PROBLEM BEHAVIOR (Code for behavior in last 7 days)
0. Behavior not exhibited in last 7 days
1. Behavior of this type occurred less than daily

SECTION D. VISION PATTERNS

1.	VISION	(Able to see in adequate light and with glasses if used)
		0. Adequate–sees fine detail, including regular print in newspapers/books
		1. Impaired – sees large print, but not regular print in newspapers/books
		2. Highly impaired – limited vision, not able to see newspaper headlines, appears to follow objects with eyes
		3. Severely impaired – no vision or appears to see only light, color, or shapes
2.	VISUAL LIMITA-TIONS/DIFF-ICULTIES	Side vision problems – decreased peripheral vision: (e.g., leaves food on one side of tray, difficulty traveling, bumps into people and objects, misjudges placement of chair when seating self) a.
		Experiences any of following: sees halos or rings around lights, sees flashes of light; sees "curtains" over eyes b.
		NONE OF ABOVE c.
3.	VISUAL APPLIANCES	Glasses; contact lenses; lens implant; magnifying glass
		0. No 1. Yes

SOUTH DAKOTA MDS+ 12/1/90B

2.		Behavior of this type occurred daily or more frequently
		a. WANDERING (moved with no rational purpose; seemingly oblivious to needs or safety)
		b. VERBALLY ABUSIVE (others were threatened, screamed at, cursed at)
		c. PHYSICALLY ABUSIVE (others were hit, shoved, scratched, sexually abused)
		d. SOCIALLY INAPPROPRIATE/DISRUPTIVE BEHAVIOR (made disrupting sounds, noisy, screams, self–abusive acts, sexual behavior or disrobing in public, smeared/threw food/feces, hoarding, rummaged through others' belongings)
4.	RESIDENT RESISTS CARE	(Check all types of resistance that occurred in the last 7 days)
		Resisted taking medications/injection a.
		Resisted ADL assistance b.
		Resisted eating c.
		NONE OF ABOVE d.
5.	BEHAVIOR MANAGE-MENT PROGRAM	Behavior problem has been addressed by clinically developed behavior management program. (Note: Do not include programs that involve only physical restraints or psychotropic medications in this category.)
		0. No behavior problem
		1. Yes, addressed
		2. No, not addressed

- 2 -

Resident: _____ Date: _____ Facility: _____ Prov. No. _____

MINIMUM DATA SET PLUS FOR NURSING HOME RESIDENT ASSESSMENT AND CARE SCREENING (MDS+)
(Status in last 7 days, unless other time frame indicated)

SECTION E. CONT.

6.	CHANGE IN MOOD	Change in mood in last 90 days
		0. No change 1. Improved 2. Deteriorated
7.	CHANGE IN PROBLEM BEHAVIOR	Change in problem behavioral signs in last 90 days
		0. No change 1. Improved 2. Deteriorated

SECTION F. PSYCHOSOCIAL WELL-BEING

1.	SENSE OF INITIATIVE/ INVOLVE- MENT	At ease interacting with others	a.
		At ease doing planned or structured activities	b.
		At ease doing self-initiated activities	c.
		Establishes own goals	d.
		Pursues involvement in life of facility (e.g., makes/keeps friends; involved in group activities; responds positively to new activities; assists at religious services)	e.
		Accepts invitations into most group activities	f.
		Adjusts easily to changes in routine	g.
		NONE OF ABOVE	h.
2.	UNSETTLED RELATION- SHIPS	Covert/open conflict with and/or repeated criticism of staff	a.
		Unhappy with roommate	b.
		Unhappy with residents other than roommate	c.
		Openly expresses conflict/anger with family or friends	d.
		Absence of personal contact with family/friends	e.
		Recent loss of close family member/friend	f.
		Avoids interactions with others	g.
		NONE OF ABOVE	h.
3.	PAST ROLES	Strong identification with past roles and life status	a.
		Expresses sadness/anger/empty feeling over lost roles/status	b.
		NONE OF ABOVE	c.

5.	PREFERS MORE OR DIFFERENT ACTIVITIES	Resident expresses/indicates preferences for other activities/choices.
		0. No 1. Yes
6.	ISOLATION ORDERS	Resident is under medical orders for isolation which prohibits participation in group activities.
		0. No 1. Yes

SECTION H. PHYSICAL FUNCTIONING AND STRUCTURAL PROBLEMS

1.	ADL SELF-PERFORMANCE		1	2
	(Code for resident's PERFORMANCE OVER ALL SHIFTS during last 7 days - not including setup)		S e l f	S u p p o r t
	0. INDEPENDENT – No help or oversight – OR – Help/oversight provided only 1 or 2 times during last 7 days.			
	1. SUPERVISION – Oversight, encouragement or cueing provided 3+ times during last 7 days – OR – Supervision plus physical assistance provided only 1 or 2 times during last 7 days.			
	2. LIMITED ASSISTANCE – Resident highly involved in activity; received physical help in guided maneuvering of limbs, or other nonweight bearing assistance 3+ times – OR – More help provided only 1 or 2 times during last 7 days.			
	3. EXTENSIVE ASSISTANCE – While resident performed part of activity, over last 7-day period, help of following type(s) provided 3 or more times:			
	– Weight-bearing support			
	– Full staff performance during part (but not all) of last 7 days			
	4. TOTAL DEPENDENCE – Full staff performance of activity during ENTIRE 7 days.			
2.	ADL SUPPORT PROVIDED -- (Code for MOST SUPPORT PROVIDED OVER ALL SHIFTS during last 7 days; code regardless of resident's self-performance classification)			
	0. No setup or physical help from staff			

SECTION G. ACTIVITY PURSUIT PATTERNS

1.	TIME AWAKE	(Check appropriate time periods over last 7 days) Resident awake all or most of time (i.e., naps no more than one hour per time period) in the:
		Morning a. Evening c.
		Afternoon b. NONE OF ABOVE d.
2.	AVERAGE TIME INVOLVED IN ACTIVITIES	0. Most (more than 2/3 of time)
		1. Some (between 1/3 and 2/3 of time)
		2. Little (less than 1/3 of time)
		3. None
3.	PREFERRED ACTIVITY SETTINGS	(Check all settings in which activities are preferred)
		Own room a. Outside facility d.
		Day/activities room b. NONE OF ABOVE e.
		Inside NH/off unit c.
4.	GENERAL ACTIVITIES PREFERENCES (Adapted to resident's current abilities)	(Check all PREFERENCES whether or not activity is currently available to resident)
		Cards/other games a. Trips/shopping g.
		Crafts/arts b. Walking/wheeling outdoors h.
		Exercise/sports c. Watch TV i.
		Music d. Gardening/plants j.
		Read/write e. Talking/conversing k.
		Spiritual/religious activities f. Helping others l.
		NONE OF ABOVE m.

1. Setup help only
2. One-person physical assist
3. Two + persons physical assist

			P r f	o r t
a.	BED MOBILITY	How resident moves to and from lying position, turns side to side, and positions body while in bed		
b.	TRANSFER	How resident moves between surfaces – to/from: bed, chair, wheelchair, standing position (EXCLUDE to/from bath/toilet)		
c.	LOCO-MOTION	How resident moves between locations in his/her room and adjacent corridor on same floor. If in wheelchair, self-sufficiency once in chair		
d.	DRESSING	How resident puts on, fastens, and takes off all items of street clothing, including donning/removing prosthesis		
e.	EATING	How resident eats and drinks (regardless of skill)		
f.	TOILET USE	How resident uses the toilet room (or commode, bedpan, urinal); tranfers on/off toilet, cleanses, changes pad, manages ostomy or catheter, adjusts clothes		
g.	PERSONAL HYGIENE	How resident maintains personal hygiene, including combing hair, brushing teeth, shaving, applying makeup, washing/drying face, hands, and perineum (EXCLUDE baths and showers)		

SOUTH DAKOTA MDS+ 12/1/90B

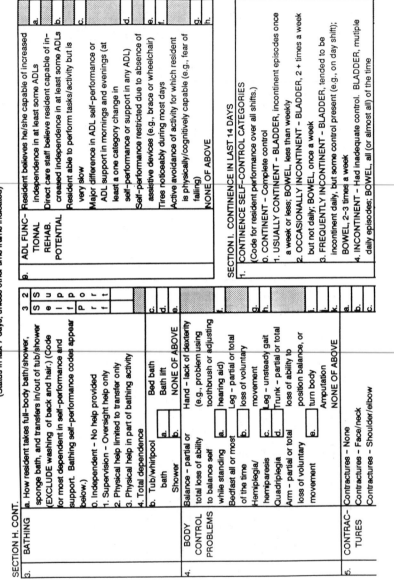

Resident: _____   Date: _____   Facility: _____   Prov. No. _____

MINIMUM DATA SET PLUS FOR NURSING HOME RESIDENT ASSESSMENT AND CARE SCREENING (MDS+)
(Status in last 7 days, unless other time frame indicated)

SECTION H. CONT.

3. BATHING

a. How resident takes full-body bath/shower, sponge bath, and transfers in/out of tub/shower (EXCLUDE washing of back and hair.) (Code for most dependent in self-performance and support. Bathing self-performance codes appear below.)

0. Independent – No help provided
1. Supervision – Oversight help only
2. Physical help limited to transfer only
3. Physical help in part of bathing activity
4. Total dependence

(columns: 3 2 / S S e u l p p o r r f f t)

b. Tub/whirlpool bath ... Bed bath
   Shower ... Bath lift
   NONE OF ABOVE

4. BODY CONTROL PROBLEMS

a. Balance – partial or total loss of ability to balance self while standing
b. Bedfast all or most of the time
c. Hemiplegia/ hemiparesis
d. Quadriplegia
e. Arm – partial or total loss of voluntary movement
   Hand – lack of dexterity (e.g., problem using toothbrush or adjusting hearing aid)
   Leg – partial or total loss of voluntary movement
   Leg – unsteady gait
   Trunk – partial or total loss of ability to position balance, or turn body
   Amputation
   NONE OF ABOVE

5. CONTRACTURES

a. Contractures – None
b. Contractures – Face/neck
c. Contractures – Shoulder/elbow

9. ADL FUNCTIONAL REHAB. POTENTIAL

a. Resident believes he/she capable of increased independence in at least some ADLs
b. Direct care staff believe resident capable of increased independence in at least some ADLs
c. Resident able to perform tasks/activity but is very slow
d. Major difference in ADL self-performance or ADL support in mornings and evenings (at least a one category change in self-performance or support in any ADL)
e. Self-performance restricted due to absence of assistive devices (e.g., brace or wheelchair)
f. Tires noticeably during most days
g. Active avoidance of activity for which resident is physically/cognitively capable (e.g., fear of falling)
h. NONE OF ABOVE

SECTION I. CONTINENCE IN LAST 14 DAYS

1. CONTINENCE SELF-CONTROL CATEGORIES (Code for resident performance over all shifts.)

0. CONTINENT – Complete control
1. USUALLY CONTINENT – BLADDER, incontinent episodes once a week or less; BOWEL, less than weekly
2. OCCASIONALLY INCONTINENT – BLADDER, 2 + times a week but not daily; BOWEL, once a week
3. FREQUENTLY INCONTINENT – BLADDER, tended to be incontinent daily, but some control present (e.g., on day shift); BOWEL, 2-3 times a week
4. INCONTINENT – Had inadequate control. BLADDER, mutiple daily episodes; BOWEL, all (or almost all) of the time

Contractures - Hand/wrist — d.
Contractures - Hip/knee — e.
Contractures - Foot/ankle — f.

6. MOBILITY APPLIANCES / DEVICES
Cane/Walker — a.
Brace/Prosthesis — b.
Wheeled self — c.
Other person wheeled — d.
Lifted (manually/mechanically) — e.
Transfer aid (slide brd) — f.
Trapeze — g.
NONE OF ABOVE — h.

7. TASK SEG-MENTATION — Resident requires that some or all of ADL activities be broken into a series of sub-tasks so that resident can perform them.
0. No.   1. Yes

8. CHANGE IN ADL SELF - PER-FORMANCE — Change in ADL self performance in last 90 days
0. No change   1. Improved   2. Deteriorated

a. BOWEL CONTI-NENCE — Control of bowel movement, with appliance or bowel continence programs, if employed

b. BLADDER CONTI-NENCE — Control of urinary bladder function (if dribbles, volume insufficient to soak through underpants), with appliances (e.g., foley) or continence programs, if employed

2. INCONTI-NENCE RELATED TESTING — (Skip if resident's bladder and bowel continence codes equal 0 / 1 and no catheter used)
Resident has been tested for a urinary tract infection — a.
Resident has been checked for presence of a fecal impaction — b.
There is adequate bowel elimination — c.
NONE OF ABOVE — d.

3. APPLIANCES AND PROGRAMS
Any scheduled toilet-ing plan — a.
External (condom) catheter — b.
Indwelling catheter — c.
Intermittent catheter — d.
Did not use toilet rm/commode/urinal — e.
Pads/briefs used — f.
Enemas/irrigation — g.
Ostomy — h.
NONE OF ABOVE — i.

4. CHANGE IN URINARY CONTI-NENCE — Change in urinary continence/appliances or programs in last 90 days
0. No change   1. Improved   2. Deteriorated

- 4 -

Resident: _____ Date: _____ Facility: _____ Prov. No. _____

MINIMUM DATA SET PLUS FOR NURSING HOME RESIDENT ASSESSMENT AND CARE SCREENING (MDS+)
(Status in last 7 days, unless other time frame indicated)

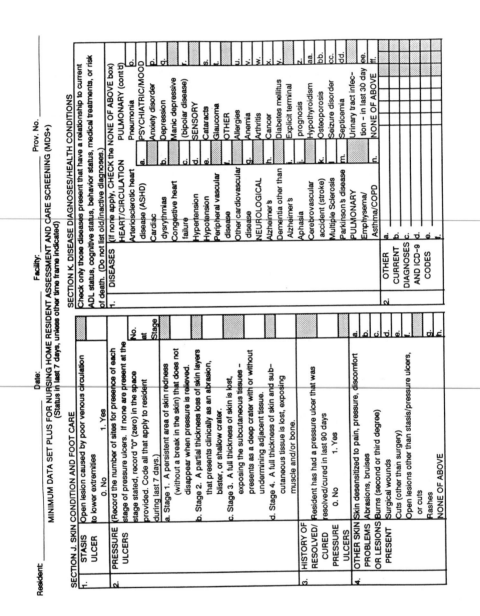

SECTION J. SKIN CONDITION AND FOOT CARE

1. STASIS ULCER — Open lesion caused by poor venous circulation to lower extremities.
0. No 1. Yes

2. PRESSURE ULCERS (Record the number of sites for presence of each stage of pressure ulcers. If none are present at the stage stated, record "0" (zero) in the space provided. Code all that apply to resident during last 7 days.)

No. at Stage

a. Stage 1. A persistent area of skin redness (without a break in the skin) that does not disappear when pressure is relieved.

b. Stage 2. A partial thickness loss of skin layers that presents clinically as an abrasion, blister, or shallow crater.

c. Stage 3. A full thickness of skin is lost, exposing the subcutaneous tissues – presents as a deep crater with or without undermining adjacent tissue.

d. Stage 4. A full thickness of skin and sub-cutaneous tissue is lost, exposing muscle and/or bone.

3. HISTORY OF RESOLVED/CURED PRESSURE ULCERS — Resident has had a pressure ulcer that was resolved/cured in last 90 days.
0. No 1. Yes

4. OTHER SKIN PROBLEMS OR LESIONS PRESENT
a. Skin desensitized to pain, pressure, discomfort
b. Abrasions, bruises
c. Burns (second or third degree)
d. Surgical wounds
e. Cuts (other than surgery)
f. Open lesions other than stasis/pressure ulcers, or cuts
g. Rashes
h. NONE OF ABOVE

SECTION K. DISEASE DIAGNOSES/HEALTH CONDITIONS

Check only those diseases present that have a relationship to current ADL status, cognitive status, behavior status, medical treatments, or risk of death. (Do not list old/inactive diagnoses.)

1. DISEASES (If none apply, CHECK the NONE OF ABOVE box)

HEART/CIRCULATION
a. Arteriosclerotic heart disease (ASHD)
b. Cardiac dysrhythmias
c. Congestive heart failure
d. Hypertension
e. Hypotension
f. Peripheral vascular disease
g. Other cardiovascular disease

NEUROLOGICAL
h. Alzheimer's
i. Dementia other than Alzheimer's
j. Aphasia
k. Cerebrovascular accident (stroke)
l. Multiple Sclerosis
m. Parkinson's disease

PULMONARY
n. Emphysema/Asthma/COPD

PULMONARY (cont'd)
o. Pneumonia

PSYCHIATRIC/MOOD
p. Anxiety disorder
q. Depression
r. Manic depressive (bipolar disease)

SENSORY
s. Cataracts
t. Glaucoma

OTHER
u. Allergies
v. Anemia
w. Arthritis
x. Cancer
y. Diabetes mellitus
z. Explicit terminal prognosis
aa. Hypothyroidism
bb. Osteoporosis
cc. Seizure disorder
dd. Septicemia
ee. Urinary tract infection – in last 30 day
ff. NONE OF ABOVE

2. OTHER CURRENT DIAGNOSES AND ICD-9 CODES
a.
b.
c.
d.
e.
f.

5.	ACTIVE SKIN CARE PROGRAM	Preventive/Protective Skin Care	a.
		Turning/repositioning program	b.
		Pressure relieving beds, bed/chair pads (e. g., egg crate pads)	c.
		Surgical wound or pressure ulcer care	d.
		Other skin care/treatment	e.
		Special nutrition/hydration program	f.
		Special application/ointments/medications	g.
		Ostomy care (e.g., trach) (routine/stable)	h.
		NONE OF ABOVE	i.
6.	SPECIAL STOCKINGS	During the last 7 days has the resident used TED or similar stockings? 0. No 1. Yes	
7.	FOOT CARE	(Check all that apply to resident during LAST 30 DAYS)	
		Preventive/Protective Foot Care (e.g., special shoes, inserts, pads, toe separators, nail/callus trimming, etc.)	a.
		Active Foot Care Treatments: Foot soaks	b.
		Dressing with and without topical medications, etc.	c.
		NONE OF ABOVE	d.

3.	PROBLEMS/ CONDITIONS AND SIGNS/ SYMPTOMS	(Check all that are present in last 7 days, UNLESS OTHER TIME FRAME INDICATED)			
		Constipation	a.	Recurrent lung aspirations in last 90 days	j.
		Diarrhea	b.	Shortness of breath (Dyspnea)	k.
		Dizziness/ vertigo	c.	Syncope (fainting)	l.
		Fecal impaction	d.	Vomiting	m.
		Fever	e.	Respiratory infection	n.
		Hallucinations/ delusions	f.	Chest Pain	o.
		Internal bleeding	g.	NONE OF ABOVE	p.
		Joint pain	h.		
		Pain – Res. com- plains or shows evidence of pain daily or almost daily	i.		
4.	EDEMA	(Check all that apply in the last 7 days)			
		Edema – none	a.		
		Edema – generalized	b.		
		Edema – localized not pitting	c.		
		Edema – pitting	d.		
		Edema – other	e.		

SOUTH DAKOTA MDS+ 12/1/90B

Resident: _____ Date: _____ Facility: _____ Prov. No. _____

48 O B R A I m p l e m e n t a t i o n

MINIMUM DATA SET PLUS FOR NURSING HOME RESIDENT ASSESSMENT AND CARE SCREENING (MDS+)
(Status in last 7 days, unless other time frame indicated)

SECTION K. CONT.

5.	ACCIDENTS	Fell – past 30 days	a.
		Fell – past 31–180 days	b.
		Hip fracture in last 180 days	a.
		last 180 days	b.
		Other fractures in last 180 days	c.
		NONE OF ABOVE	d.

6.	STABILITY OF CONDITIONS	Conditions/diseases make resident's cognitive, ADL, or behavior status unstable–fluctuating, precarious, or deteriorating.	a.
		Resident experiencing an acute episode or a flare-up of a recurrent/chronic problem.	b.
		NONE OF ABOVE	c.

SECTION L. ORAL/NUTRITIONAL STATUS

1.	ORAL PROBLEMS	Chewing problem	a.
		Swallowing problem	b.
		Mouth pain	c.
		NONE OF ABOVE	d.

2.	HEIGHT AND WEIGHT	a. Record height in inches	HT (in.)
		b. Record weight in pounds	WT (lb.)
		Weight based on most recent status in last 30 days; measure weight consistently in accord with standard facility practice – e.g., in a.m. after voiding before meal, with shoes off, and in nightclothes.	
		c. Weight loss (i.e., 5% plus IN THE PAST 30 DAYS or 10% IN THE PAST 180 DAYS):	
		0. No 1. Yes	

SECTION M. ORAL/DENTAL STATUS

1.	ORAL STATUS AND DISEASE PREVENTION	Debris (soft, easily movable substances) present in mouth prior to going to bed at night	a.
		Has dentures and/or removable bridge	b.
		Some/all natural teeth lost – does not have or does not use dentures (or partial plates)	c.
		Broken, loose, or carious teeth	d.
		Inflamed gums (gingiva); swollen or bleeding gums; oral abscesses, ulcers, or rashes	e.
		Daily cleaning of teeth/dentures	f.
		NONE OF ABOVE	g.

SECTION N. SPECIAL TREATMENTS, DEVICES, PROC., & SUPPLIES

1.	SPECIAL TREAT-MENTS AND PRO-CEDURES	a. SPECIAL CARE – (Check treatments received during the last 14 days.)	
		Chemotherapy	a.
		Radiation	b.
		Dialysis	c.
		Suctioning	d.
		Trach care	e.
		IV meds.	f.
		Transfusions	g.
		O2	h.
		Intake/Output	i.
		Ventilator/Respirator	j.
		Other	k.
		NONE OF ABOVE	

b. THERAPIES – Record the number of days and total minutes each of these therapies was administered (for at least 10 minutes) in the last 7 days (0 if none)
Box A = # of days administered for 10 min.s or more administered in last 7 days
Box B = Total # of minutes administered in last 7 days

		A	B
a.	Speech – language pathology and audiology services		
b.	Occupational therapy		
c.	Physical therapy		
d.	Psychological therapy (any lic. prof.)		

3.	NUTRITIONAL PROBLEMS	Complains about the taste of many foods	a.	Regular complaint of hunger
		Insufficient fluid; dehydrated	b.	Leaves 25% + food uneaten at most meals
		Did NOT consume all/almost all liquids provided during last 3 days	c.	NONE OF ABOVE

4.	NUTRITIONAL APPROACHES	Parenteral/IV	a.	Therapeutic diet
		Feeding tube	b.	Dietary supplement between meals
		Mechanically altered diet	c.	Plate guard, stabilized built-up utensil, etc.
		Syringe (oral feeding)	d.	NONE OF ABOVE

| | | e. Respiratory therapy |
| | | f. Recreation therapy |

2.	REHABILITATION/RESTORATIVE CARE	Record the NUMBER OF DAYS each of the following rehabilitation/restorative technique/practice was provided for more than or equal to 15 minutes per day to the resident in the last 7 days. (Enter 0 if none)
		a. Range of Motion (passive)
		b. Range of Motion (active)
		c. Splint/Brace Assistance
		d. Reality Orientation
		e. Remotivation
		Training and Skill Practice in:
		f. Locomotion/Mobility
		g. Dressing/Grooming
		h. Eating/Swallowing
		i. Transfer
		j. Amputation care

3.	DEVICES AND RESTRAINTS	Use the following code for last 7 days:
		0. Not used
		1. Used less than daily
		2. Used daily
		a. Bed rails
		b. Trunk restraint
		c. Limb restraint
		d. Chair prevents rising

Resident: _____ Date: _____ Facility: _____ Prov. No. _____

MINIMUM DATA SET PLUS FOR NURSING HOME RESIDENT ASSESSMENT AND CARE SCREENING (MDS+)
(Status in last 7 days, unless other time frame indicated)

SECTION N. CONT.

4.	SUPPLIES	Record the number of units of the supply listed that have been used or consumed by the resident in the past 7 days. (Enter 0 if none)
		a. Sterile Dressings
		b. Unique/Special Decubitus Care Supplies
		c. Peritoneal Dialysis Supplies
5.	PHYSICIAN VISITS / ORDERS	IN THE PRIOR 30-DAY PERIOD / since the resident was admitted, how many times has the physician (authorized assistant/practitioner) changed the resident's orders? (Do not include order renewals without change).
6.	NO LAB TEST	Check if no laboratory tests performed in last 90 days. (Skip to Section O.) a.
7.	LABORATORY TEST	How many lab samples (blood/urine/etc.) have been collected IN THE PAST 30 DAYS?
8.	ABNORMAL LAB RESULTS	a. How many laboratory tests were returned with abnormal values during the past 90 days?
		b. How many abnormal values resulted in treatment or care planning in the past 30 days?

SECTION O. MEDICATION USE

1.	NUMBER OF MEDICATIONS	Record the number of different medications used in the last 7 days; (enter "0" if none used. Skip to Item 5.)
2.	NEW MEDICATIONS	Resident has received new medication during the last 90 days. 0. No 1. Yes
3.	INJECTIONS	Record the number of days injections of any type received during the last 7 days.
4.	DAYS RECEIVED THE FOLLOWING MEDICATION	Record the NUMBER OF DAYS during the last 7 days; enter "0" if not used; enter "1" if long-acting meds. used less than weekly.
		a. Antipsychotics
		b. Antianxiety/hypnotics
		c. Antidepressants
5.	PREVIOUS MEDICATION RESULTS	Skip this question if resident currently receiving antipsychotics, antidepressants, or antianxiety/hypnotics – otherwise code correct response for last 90 days.
		Resident has previously received psychoactive medications for a mood or behavior problem, and these medications were effective (without undue adverse consequences).
		0. No, drugs not used
		1. Drugs were effective
		2. Drugs were not effective
		3. Drug effectiveness unknown

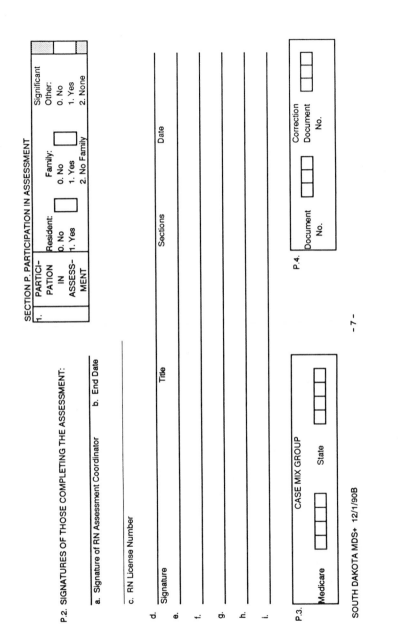

SECTION P. PARTICIPATION IN ASSESSMENT

1.	PARTICI-PATION IN ASSESS-MENT	Resident: 0. No 1. Yes	Family: 0. No 1. Yes 2. No Family	Significant Other: 0. No 1. Yes 2. None

P.2. SIGNATURES OF THOSE COMPLETING THE ASSESSMENT:

a. Signature of RN Assessment Coordinator   b. End Date

c. RN License Number

	Signature	Title	Sections	Date
d.				
e.				
f.				
g.				
h.				
i.				

P.3. CASE MIX GROUP

Medicare   State

P.4. Document No.   Correction Document No.

SOUTH DAKOTA MDS+ 12/1/90B

- 7 -

Resident: _____ Date: _____ Facility: _____ Prov. No. _____

SOUTH DAKOTA

MINIMUM DATA SET PLUS FOR NURSING HOME RESIDENT ASSESSMENT AND CARE SCREENING (MDS+)
(Status in last 7 days unless other time frame indicated)

SECTION Q. MEDICATIONS LIST

List all medications given during the last 7 days. Include medications used regularly less than weekly as part of the resident's treatment regimen.

1. List the medication name and the dosage

2. RA (Route of Administration). Use the appropriate code from the following list:

   1 = by mouth (PO)
   2 = sublingual (SL)
   3 = intramuscular (IM)
   4 = intravenous (IV)
   5 = subcutaneous (SubQ)
   6 = rectally
   7 = topical
   8 = inhalation
   9 = enteral tube
   10 = other

3. FREQ (Frequency): Use appropriate frequency code to show the number of times per day that the medication was given.

   PR = (PRN) as necessary
   1H = (qh) every hour
   2H = (q2h) every two hours
   3H = (q3h) every three hours
   4H = (q4h) every four hours
   6H = (q6h) every six hours
   8H = (q8h) every eight hours
   1D = (qd or hs) once daily

   2D = (BID) two times daily
      (includes every 12 hours)
   3D = (TID) three times daily
   4D = (QID) four times daily
   5D = five times a day
   1W = (QWeek) once every week
   2W = twice every week
   3W = three times every week

   QO = every other day
   4W = four times every week
   5W = five times every week
   6W = six times every week
   1M = (QMonth) once every month
   2M = twice every month
   C = continuous

4. PRN-n (prn-number of doses): If the frequency code is "PR", record the number of times during the past 7 days that each PRN medication was given. Do not use this column for scheduled medications.

5. DRUG CODE: Enter the National Drug Code (NDC).

NOTE: If using the NDC's in the Manual Appendix

The last two digits of the 11 digit NDC define package size and have been omitted from the codes listed in the Manual Appendix. If using this Appendix, the NDC should be entered left-justified (the first digit of the code should be entered in the space farthest to the left of the NDC code column). This should result in the last two spaces being left blank.

1. Medication Name and Dosage	2. RA	3. Freq	4. PRN-n	NDC Codes
EXAMPLE: Coumadin 2.5mg	1	1W		
Digoxin 0.125 mg	1	1D		
Humulin R 25 Units	5	1D		
Robitussin 15cc	1	PR	2	

Resident: _____ Date: _____ Facility: _____ Prov. No. _____

SOUTH DAKOTA

MINIMUM DATA SET PLUS FOR NURSING HOME RESIDENT ASSESSMENT AND CARE SCREENING (MDS+)
(Status in last 7 days unless other time frame indicated)

1. Medication Name and Dosage	2. RA	3. Freq	4. PRN-n	NDC Codes

United Hebrew Geriatric Center: Restraint Policy

Neil Dworkin and Patricia McCormack

THE OBRA mandate of 1987 challenged long-term care facilities throughout the United States to enact vigorous restraint minimization programs. The New York State Department of Health (NYSDOH 1992) considers restraint use to be a gross insult to residents' sense of worth and autonomy. It emphasizes the need for a comprehensive interdisciplinary assessment focusing on the distinguishing features and competencies of the individual resident concerned. Restraint-free care should be achieved by a series of planned strategies identifying steps towards the desired outcome. Facilities have been advised against arbitrarily removing restraints without proper planning based on measurable goals and objectives. Given the right to be an active member of the care planning process, the resident or his or her designated representative must not be coerced into accepting a restraint, even if it is deemed appropriate for his or her well-being by hospital or nursing home staff.

Federal and state regulatory agencies have made restraint issues a major priority for ongoing surveillance in all long-term care facilities. Compliance is monitored through the patient review instrument (PRI), which is submitted at regular intervals for reimbursement purposes. Similarly, the Minimum Data Set, a comprehensive interdisciplinary assessment tool mandated by OBRA, includes indicators of restraint use. These data sources provide surveyors with information about resident care issues, including restraint use, prior to their visits.

This case is based on the authors' experience implementing a restraint minimization program at the United Hebrew Geriatric Center in New Rochelle, New York.

Surveyors view restraints as indicators of negative quality of life. In assessing cases in which restraints have been used, they scrutinize the resident's behavior, and review supporting documentation, care planning, and alternatives previously tried. A physician's order alone is not an adequate criterion to justify restraint use as a care modality.

Restraint Minimization at UHGC

The Restraint Minimization Program at the United Hebrew Geriatric Center (UHGC) was based on the New York State Nursing Home Code (415.2). New York State Code 415.13 defines a physical restraint as:

> Any manual method or physical or mechanical device, material, or equipment attached or adjacent to the resident's body, that the individual cannot remove easily, which restricts freedom of movement or normal access to one's body, which are used only to protect the health and safety of the resident and to assist the resident to attain and maintain optimum levels of physical and emotional functioning.

Prior to introducing the restraint minimization program in UHGC's four skilled nursing units, approximately 40 percent of 166 residents were in some form of restraint. Their ages ranged from 70–107 years, with a mean of 88 years. The vast majority suffered from multiple chronic conditions associated with old age, including heart disease, chronic obstructive pulmonary disease, arthritis, Parkinsonism, diabetes mellitus, and organic brain syndrome. They also were severely impaired in functioning, related to diminished intellect and judgment, visual and hearing deficits, and incontinence. In addition, many manifested varying degrees of physical frailty, placing them at a high risk of falling. Fully 75 percent of residents required some degree of assistance with transfers and locomotion. The remaining 25 percent required a two-person lift for in- and out-of-bed maneuvers.

Three of the skilled units have 40 residents each, and one has 46. The Intensive Therapeutic Care Unit, Unit 3, specializes in care of residents afflicted with Alzheimer's disease. Manifestations of this condition range from disorganized thinking to severe behavioral aberrations, including verbal disruption, combativeness, and antisocial actions.

As of two years ago, having already reduced restraint use from 46 to 34 percent, administrative staff from UHGC and 21 other facilities in the region were summoned to the NYSDOH local office and advised that their prevailing restraint practices were unacceptable. PRI data, illustrating quality of life triggers, including restraint use, were presented. It ranked each facility, anonymously, in terms of restraints and other critical care issues.

Following the meeting, it was clear that the UHGC staff had to re-think their prior restraint minimization strategy. Existing policy, reflected in the mission statement, affirmed the Nursing Home Code (NYCRR 415.4) position on restraint use:

> Quality of life, which encompasses dignity, independence, freedom of move-ment, and autonomy epitomizes the mission of the United Hebrew Geriatric Center. Therefore, minimal restraint usage will be the standard of care for our residents. Restraint management shall only be utilized when all other measures to assure resident safety have been exhausted.

As part of the new restraint minimization program residents were reassessed using an interdisciplinary team approach. The goal was to have no more than 5 percent of residents restrained. Nursing staff on all shifts, including certified nurse attendants, the first line caregivers, were involved in selecting residents to participate. Each week one or two residents on each unit were placed on the minimization program. A policy was formulated outlining each step of the process. Family and physician consent was obtained prior to the initiation of any restraint minimization program. Input from nursing staff served as the basis for the restraint minimization care plan process, and was finalized in an Interdisciplinary Care Plan meeting. The plan clearly identified the hours when the resident would be restraint-free. One of the major positive results of the program was the increased sensitivity of staff to residents' needs and greater understanding of the range of restraint alternatives for resident safety and behavior control.

Restraint alternatives included positioning devices such as cushions, lateral supports, reclining wheelchairs, and self-release belts. Restrain-ing geri-chairs were discontinued and geri-reclining chairs were outfit-ted with positioning devices based on resident need. Other strategies included "Unit Walkathons" for agitated and wandering residents. A "My Time" group was established for severely disruptive residents on the Alzheimer's unit, taking them off the unit to a quiet room twice daily for two-and-a-half hours each session. Finally, with funds from the Ladies' Auxiliary, art therapy students from a local college began to run a program with residents, assisting them with self-expression through various projects.

Restraint Reduction and Accident Data

Figures 3.1 and 3.2 depict the progress achieved under the Restraint Minimization Program. Restraints have been reduced from the high of 46 percent in 1990, and 34 percent in 1992, to 5 percent in 1994. Despite reports in the literature suggesting reduced accidents resulting from restraint reduction (Blakeslee et al. 1991), accidents at UHGC doubled in the first two years of the program. While minor injuries sustained increased almost three-fold, major injuries such as bone fracture, declined by one-third. Further study is needed to determine the extent to which the accidents were caused by falls and whether the rate has subsequently declined.

The Case of Mr. Greene

Mr. Greene has been a resident of the Intensive Therapeutic Care unit for six months. At age 78, his diagnoses include multiple-infarct dementia and a history of seizure disorder. He has a marked visual deficit and is legally blind. His speech, hearing, and fine motor skills are essentially intact. Mr. Greene's ambulatory skills fluctuate from independent to needing assistance from one person, according to his mental status. He is disoriented to time and place and displays diminished judgment and safety awareness. Mr. Greene also wanders, wanting to go home, frequently going to the elevator.

According to nursing staff on all three shifts, Mr. Greene's behavioral aberrations include from mild to severe verbal disruption and physical aggression. Regular weeping appears to be brought on by "life review" of painful experiences, including probable physical and sexual abuse as a

Figure 3.1 Restraint Minimization: Residents in Restraints out of 163

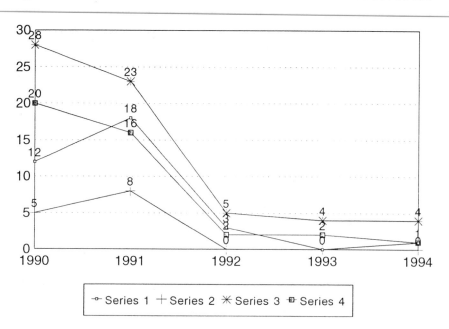

Figure 3.2   Accidents and Injuries by Unit

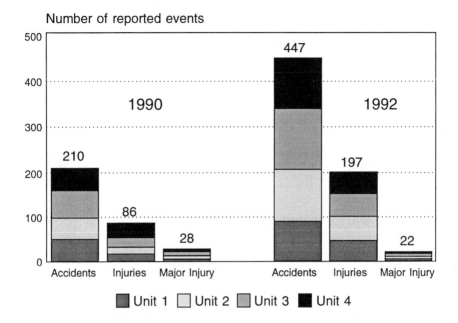

child. His verbal abuse and combative behavior are common during staff interviews and aggressive overtones are prevalent during care routines. For example, Mr. Greene hits, bites, kicks, and pushes caregivers; approaching him for any reason is a challenge. Mr. Greene is clearly at high risk for falls. During an eight-week period, he sustained eight falls, none resulting in serious injury. He also manifests a propensity for injury to self and others because of his unpredictable aggression and wandering.

Care of Mr. Greene

Following medical and psychiatric assessment, various psychotropic medications were administered, starting with a minimum dose, in an attempt to reduce his agitation. After four weeks of therapy, medications were discontinued because he continued weeping, was increasingly lethargic, and showed no discernible change in other behaviors. He is presently receiving antidepressant medication, the efficacy of which remains to be determined.

Concurrently with drug therapy, intervention by nursing staff focused on maximizing Mr. Greene's safety while allowing him as much freedom of movement as possible. Conferences were conducted with his family and various staff disciplines. It was decided that Mr. Greene would be placed in a reclining geri-chair on an emergency basis, only when he was extremely agitated. When Mr. Greene made several attempts to climb over the back of the chair, use of an upright geri-chair with a tray was instituted.

A plan of care was developed outlining specific restraint time periods and non-restraint time activities. The plan requires ongoing adjustment due to Mr. Greene's unpredictable behavior. Its goal is to have him restrained for no more than six to eight hours in any 24 hour period.

Nursing staff continued to allow Mr. Greene as much freedom of movement as was practicable. He is permitted supervised ambulation on and off the unit if his gait is steady and he is nonaggressive. He attends a two-and-one-half hour session of the "My Time" group, unrestrained, each afternoon that his behavior permits. He is also included in unit programs when he is receptive to participation.

During the night shift, a certified nursing attendant sits outside his door. His sleep is very poor; he generally sleeps only one night out of four. Medication has not been effective in this area. Staff report that Mr. Greene is typically awake during the early part of the night. When he is in a regular chair, he constantly reaches to the floor. If he is returned to bed when agitated, his emotional situation escalates. When extremely agitated at night, Mr. Greene is placed in a geri-chair with a tray in front of the nurses' station. He is ambulated every two hours for fifteen minutes. Towards dawn, he becomes drowsy and is placed in bed, but appears to be tormented by nightmares. He is permitted to sleep late in the morning because of his poor sleep, and is served breakfast when he awakens.

Thus far, nursing strategies have not been successful in significantly minimizing Mr. Greene's restraint use. Staff constantly review his status and maintain a goal of his becoming restraint-free. Mr. Greene is one of several residents frustrating staff efforts toward becoming a restraint-free facility.

Conclusion

The Restraint Minimization Program at UHGC is an unfinished effort. There is no doubt that the quality of life of a resident freed of restraint is greatly enhanced. The challenge and ultimate goal is to have a wholly restraint-free environment—an ideal which has been achieved by other facilities and can be achieved at UHGC in the future. This process will require ongoing multidisciplinary teamwork and creativity, and must be linked to the consistent application of policies and procedures, monitoring forms, staff education, and family involvement, in an effort to provide the best possible quality of life for residents. Staff now have to develop a plan to complete the job of creating a restraint-free environment at UHGC.

References

Blakeslee, J. A., B. D. Goldman, D. Papougenis, and C. A. Torell. 1991. "Making the Transition to Restraint-Free Care." *Gerontological Nursing* (February).

New York State Code of Rules and Regulations. 1990. Chapter 5, "Medical Facilities, Subchapter A, Minimum Standards, Article 3, Residential Care Facilities." Part 415, Nursing Home Minimum Standards.

New York State Department of Health. 1992. Published memorandum series 92–13, "Nursing Home Resident Rights." January.

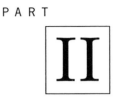
Quality Assurance and
Quality Improvement

The Fenway Nursing and Convalescent Center: Maggots in Decubiti

James E. Allen

THE SECRETARY of the Massachusetts Department of Health phoned Amy Baxter, the director of Health Services, just as Amy was finishing her second cup of coffee. The secretary had just read the front page nursing home story in the Sunday edition of the *Boston News*. He told Amy that while he had no control over June Sheffield R.N. because she was a federal Medicare inspector, he thought he must have some control over Massachusetts officials. He had talked at length earlier that morning with Jane O'Brien, the social worker who was pressing for a criminal investigation into the Cohen case. In wrapping up the call he told Amy to put together a succinct memo summarizing what the state's position should be on the culpability of the nursing facility where Dr. Cohen stayed before her leg was amputated. He wanted it on his desk by next Friday morning at the latest because he expected to hear from irate citizens from the Boston and Brookline areas.

Ms. Baxter placed some phone calls and read up on the Cohen case. The following is a summary of her findings on the events that led to the early Sunday morning call from the secretary of health.

Background

Dr. Cohen was an 89-year-old resident of Fenway Nursing and Convalescent Center (FNCC), located on Babcock Street in Brookline, a

The care information and activities in this case are based on real events. The names of people and the facility have been changed.

well-to-do suburb adjoining Boston. Dr. Cohen had been a successful local physician, but eight years of nursing facility expenses (averaging over $30,000 per year) had depleted her life savings; she had become a Medicaid recipient two years before this incident. Dr. Cohen previously had suffered several strokes which had restricted her to a wheelchair, but her major medical problem was advancing peripheral vascular disease, involving insufficient blood circulation to the extremities.

In July, during a visit to the facility, the local ombudsperson, who had earlier befriended Dr. Cohen, saw a Stage IV decubitus ulcer on her left foot. A few days later, at 3:48 a.m., a nurse discovered and removed an infestation of maggots in the ulcer; a few weeks after that Dr. Cohen's left leg was amputated at Massachusetts General Hospital.

At the ombudsperson's request the Massachusetts Department of Social Services investigated the situation. After studying the case, two social workers, Ms. June O'Brien and Mr. Kelvin Murphy, the adult services chief, concluded that Dr. Cohen's leg had been amputated due to caretaker neglect, and sought a criminal investigation of the facility. The news story in the Boston paper was sympathetic to the ombudsperson's and the social workers' views that FNCC was criminally negligent in Dr. Cohen's care.

The Accusations

In an early-September letter regarding Dr. Cohen, Massachusetts Department of Social Services staff members O'Brien and Murphy indicated that there was clear evidence of caretaker neglect in her case. In their view, nursing facility records poorly documented Dr. Cohen's decubitus ulcer treatment and inadequately reported decubitus medical problems. Dr. Cohen's left foot decubitus lesion had been quite serious, and at one point had parasites (maggots) in the wound. O'Brien and Murphy concluded that the decubitus lesion on Dr. Cohen's heel had led to the amputation of her leg. The Health Department had helped get them access to the FNCC records, upon which they based their conclusion.

The Massachusetts State's Attorney was seeking to determine whether Fenway Nursing and Convalescent Center or any of its employees were guilty of patient abuse, criminal neglect, or both. Basic factors to be considered under this statute are whether the resident had been physically abused by any of the following that had caused serious bodily injury or death:

1. Intentional act(s)
2. Culpably negligent act(s)
3. Intentional omission(s)
4. Culpably negligent omission(s).

Findings of culpable neglect must be based on conduct of a willful, gross, and flagrant character evincing reckless disregard of human life. No nursing facility staff member had ever been found guilty under this new law. Ms. Baxter thought there were few occasions when the statutory definition of culpable negligence would be met.

Ms. Baxter suspected that Dr. Cohen's patient records, physician's reports, state and federal inspections, and state Board of Nursing reports, would not provide the degree of evidence required to prove culpable neglect. However, she thought they may indicate whether intentional or unintentional omissions occurred which could substantiate a Department of Social Services finding of caretaker neglect. By asserting that the left foot decubitus ulcer eventually led to her amputation, the Department of Social Services argued that negligent omission (not preventing or treating the lesion properly) occurred and had caused serious bodily injury.

What seemed to be O'Brien and Murphy's real question was whether Dr. Cohen had received competent health care and whether her needs had been adequately met while a resident at Fenway Nursing and Convalescent Center. In order to raise this fundamental question they had asserted the extreme position and charged neglect.

Assessment of the Quality of Care

Ms. Baxter spent most of the next five days at the Fenway Nursing and Convalescent Center gathering information for her report to the secretary of the Department of Health. Her first impression was that the caretaker neglect accusation was too general. In their report, O'Brien and Murphy simply assert caretaker neglect without citing specific examples or documenting its extent or nature from Dr. Cohen's files. Caretaker neglect seemed to be related to their assertions that there had been poor documentation and that Dr. Cohen's ulcer had resulted in an unnecessary amputation. Ms. Baxter's review of Dr. Cohen's care included review of records documenting physician care, care plans, nursing care, pharmacy needs, and personal and social needs.

Physician Care

Dr. Morales was Dr. Cohen's physician throughout her 50-month stay at Fenway. Ms. Baxter's impression from the physician's orders was that of a personal concern for Dr. Cohen's well-being. All of Dr. Morales' visits were timely and within Medicaid and Medicare guidelines. One important measure of physician concern for patients in nursing facilities is the number of telephone orders given between the Medicare mandated visits and required physician medical record updates. Table 4.1 data document Dr. Morales' telephone orders regarding Dr. Cohen's care.

Table 4.1 Telephone Orders

Years Ago	Total	Per Month
5	19	7 (3 months)
4	38	3
3	54	4
2	31	3
1	40	3

Another quality measure is the number of laboratory reports ordered by the physician. The appropriate number can be estimated from the number and types of drugs prescribed and other factors in the patient's condition or conditions. Dr. Morales ordered a total of 132 laboratory analyses, which was about the same as or slightly exceeded expectations for Dr. Cohen's conditions.

Upon notification of the ulcer, Dr. Morales ordered a new treatment regimen, which was implemented by the staff. When Dr. Cohen's ulcer failed to respond, Dr. Morales ordered a culture, again changed the treatment regimen, and called in a specialist in plastic and reconstructive surgery. The plastic surgeon gave Dr. Cohen specialized care from the fourth week after diagnosis until her hospitalization.

Dr. Cohen's necrotic toenails required appropriate professional care by a podiatrist expert in debriding necrotic nails. Between January and March, a podiatrist was called in seven times. Dr. Cohen also received care from a dentist twice each year. Physical examination records are available for each year, and her diagnosis had remained relatively stable over the multiyear period.

Plan of Care

Nursing facilities must establish a multidisciplinary plan of care to meet each resident's needs, listing problems, needs, goals, and approaches for achieving these goals for each discipline. Dr. Cohen had numerous plans of care during her stay in the facility. The plans varied appropriately as her needs and capabilities had changed over time. Each seven-page plan identified problems and needs, along with goals and approaches, in the following areas: (1) activities and socialization, (2) care of fragile skin, (3) weight maintenance, (4) management of incontinence (to minimize fragile skin breakdown), (5) dental care, (6) special care for decubitus ulcer, and (7) mobility.

Dr. Cohen's son visited two or three times each week, but less often during the winter months. The facility involved him in care planning sessions, including the one immediately prior to discovery of the decubitus ulcer, as is documented by his signature on the plan of care along with the signatures of Dr. Cohen's nurse, the activities staff member, and the dietary manager.

Nursing Care

"Condition on Admission" notes made by the admitting nurse indicated that Dr. Cohen's left toe had a blue nail with a small amount of bloody drainage. Thus, even at admission four years ago, Dr. Cohen's left foot had poor blood circulation and infection. The nurse also noted that Dr. Cohen had scars from recent decubitus ulcers on her buttocks, indicating that her peripheral vascular disease was in an advanced state. In fact, she was admitted in large part because her circulation was becoming increasingly compromised and she needed specialized skin care. At almost every monthly nursing summary staff members discussed her skin condition, and ordinarily appropriate care was successfully provided.

According to the nurses' progress notes in March, Dr. Cohen's son had wanted a catheter removed. The nurse in charge voiced a concern that removing the catheter would increase the threat to Dr. Cohen's skin integrity, so the son's request was denied.

In May of this year, the monthly nursing summary pointed out the red area around Dr. Cohen's left foot for special concern. The June report noted progress in maintaining this fragile area. In the second week of July, nursing staff noted a new decubitus ulcer and started treatment, however, treatments were not recorded for three weeks following this note.

An examination of Dr. Cohen's treatment records during her stay at FNCC indicates an awareness of Dr. Cohen's fragile skin and tracking of the ongoing care given it. However, documentation of the care given between the second and third week of July was poor. The physician had ordered the decubitus ulcer on Dr. Cohen's left foot be cleaned every shift until healed, but weekly progress reports from this period were incomplete in these areas. There was poor documentation of the use of bunny boots (soft material boots designed to spread the pressure that bony structures place on external skin areas) which the physician had ordered. Documentation of bunny boot use was complete for the 3-to-11 pm shift, but spotty on the other two shifts.

A new culture of the decubitus sore on Dr. Cohen's left foot was taken during the third week in July, and new orders subsequently given.

The new orders were documented in the treatment record as having been consistently carried out until Dr. Cohen's transfer to Massachusetts General Hospital in August.

Daily records profile Dr. Cohen's eating, bathing, ambulating, positioning, range of motion, and bowel functions. An examination of these records reveals appropriate daily care in each of these categories. She ate well and had normal bowel functions. She also received appropriate position changes to minimize skin breakdown from being in one position too long. Restraints were not used.

Vital signs flow sheets documented that Dr. Cohen had maintained her weight while at the facility, never dropping below 120 pounds. Her vital signs were appropriately recorded, her temperature, pulse, blood pressure, and weight appear to have been constantly monitored.

Similarly, decubitus flow sheets documented Dr. Cohen's decubitus ulcers over the course of her stay. She had several ulcers due to her worsening peripheral vascular disease and her fragile skin. Recent treatment to the left foot decubitus was described in a flow sheet dated July–August. Its progress from a Stage II (moderate) to a Stage IV (severe) ulcer was documented. The treatment nurse indicated the use of bunny boots to relieve pressure on sensitive skin. The nurse also noted the changes in treatment that had been prescribed by Dr. Morales.

One protection nursing facility residents receive is the legal requirement that a pharmacist review their drug regimen each month. This offers the pharmacist's opinion and evaluation of drug regimens to supplement the physician's evaluation. The pharmacist's reports over the years of Dr. Cohen's stay indicate that he monitored her treatment for drug interactions. The medical administration records (MARs) were consistently examined by the professional pharmacist, who was generally satisfied with the physician's and nurses' efforts to meet Dr. Cohen's medication needs.

Daily records were kept of the volume of liquid drank and urine excreted during each shift throughout the years of Dr. Cohen's stay at FNCC. Dehydration is a frequent reason nursing home patients end up in hospital emergency rooms. Ms. Baxter randomly picked the date of December 7 of the first year and the last year of Dr. Cohen's stay, and compared fluid levels. The results are shown in Table 4.2.

Finally, the required hospital and transfer records were also present in Dr. Cohen's files, along with a discharge plan, mandated for each resident.

Quality of Life

Because residents often live in a nursing facility for the rest of their lives, their social experiences can be as important as medical care in

Table 4.2   Dr. Cohen's Fluid Intake and Output

	Total Cubic Centimeters of Liquid	
	Dec. 7 First Year	Dec. 7 Last Year
Intake	1,010	2,340
Output	1,050	2,400

determining whether caretaker neglect has occurred. Ms. Baxter reviewed several social progress notes about Dr. Cohen's life at FNCC.

Two years ago, Dr. Cohen seemed very well-adjusted to her life at Fenway Nursing and Convalescent Center. She accepted her room and roommate, although sometimes they did get on each others' nerves. She did not have any major changes in activity and socialization during the year, and no social activity problems were reported. She attended almost every activity scheduled and enjoyed socializing with others and watching TV in her room. Her son visited often and was very supportive.

In August, the day before her transfer to the hospital, the director of Social Services talked on the telephone with Dr. Cohen's son, who said the family did not want to tell Dr. Cohen her leg would have to be amputated. The Social Services director was concerned that Dr. Cohen did not know yet, only a few days before surgery. Dr. Cohen's son wanted the doctor to explain the situation to her at the hospital. No one ever told Dr. Cohen of the impending amputation.

Exercise is important for all older persons, but especially for persons with poor blood circulation. The restorative nursing notes document that over her years of care, Dr. Cohen received daily rehabilitative exercise, with attention given to her range of motion. As might be expected, as her peripheral vascular disease worsened during the last few months of residence, her interests and ability to participate in exercise and social activities decreased commensurably. For example, in mid-March records state "the resident has to be coaxed a lot during these exercises, especially her left arm, but she does well with the games. She is being encouraged and praised for her efforts." In April, the resident "was in bed at the time of exercise class yesterday and again today." In late May, the record indicated that Dr. Cohen had to be coaxed a lot with exercises, especially when it came to using her left arm. She was always encouraged and praised for her efforts.

The dietitian followed the care and treatment of Dr. Cohen's decubitus ulcers over the years because she sought to provide dietary intake

Table 4.3   Summary of Dr. Cohen's Care

Eight years ago	Admitted to FNCC—left toe had a blue nail with bloody drainage, scars from recent decubitus ulcers on buttocks
Two years ago	Became Medicaid—Well adjusted
THIS YEAR	
Jan–March	Podiatrist called in seven times
March	Son wanted a catheter removed—denied because of threat to skin—has to be coaxed during exercises
April	In bed at time of exercises
May	Dietary notes son brings in sweet snacks—nursing concerned about red area around left foot
Late May	Had to be coaxed with exercises
June	Progress in maintaining fragile skin
Early July	Federal surveyors observed Dr. Cohen not out of bed—problems with decubitus ulcer care noted but no deficiency
July	New decubitus ulcer diagnosed—treatment begun—no treatments recorded for three weeks following this note—ulcer failed to respond, culture ordered, treatment regimen changed
Mid-July	Ombudsperson saw a Stage IV decubitus ulcer on left foot—documentation of care was poor—new culture taken—orders given and carried out
Late July	Nurse discovered and removed infestation of maggots in the ulcer
July–August	Flow sheet noted progress from Stage II to Stage IV ulcer—bunny boots used
August	Plastic surgeon provided care—transfer to Massachusetts General Hospital—amputation
Early Sept.	Letter by Department of Social Services staff—evidence of caretaker neglect
September	State survey notes too few weekly progress notes on ulcer—poor documentation of protective boot use—foot drop boot order not documented
September	State Board of Nursing found treatments were rendered and physician was notified
September	Newspaper article—call from Secretary of Health

that would promote healing. Dr. Cohen, however, preferred to eat sweets. A May dietary note reveals that Dr. Cohen's son continued to bring in snacks such as cupcakes and cookies. The son had been notified that all food should be checked in by a nurse or dietary manager. Dr. Cohen's diet order stated she was not to have sweets of any kind. The dietitian noted that she would continue to encourage the son to bring in only healthy snacks.

Survey Findings

The federal surveyors visited in July of this year. They observed that Dr. Cohen was not out of bed until the third day of the survey, even though there was no order for bedrest. They noted problems with her decubitus ulcer care, but did not believe the care merited a deficiency or a fine. Nurses and other staff indicated that Dr. Cohen was less and less mobile in the days preceding surgery.

The state conducted a survey of FNCC in early September. It reported that too few weekly progress notes had been written on Dr. Cohen's left foot decubitus ulcer. Protective boot use documentation was lacking 35 of 64 possible times. Further, use of a physician-ordered foot drop boot (a support device to maintain the foot in its normal position) was not documented.

The state Board of Nursing also inspected FNCC. In a letter to the facility, a discipline consultant concluded that during the several days for which nursing assessments had not been entered on the condition of Dr. Cohen's left foot, there was, nevertheless, documentation that the ordered treatments were being rendered. Further, the physician was appropriately notified about a change in the pressure sore in every instance.

Having completed her research, Amy Baxter summarized what she knew about the chronology of events (see Table 4.3). She now is ready to write her report for the secretary of health.

Whispering Pines Nursing and Rehabilitation Center: Implementing Corporate Total Quality Management

Henry W. Smorynski and Lois Bluhm

WHISPERING PINES Nursing and Rehabilitation Center (WPNRC) is a 220-bed facility located in Tarleton Springs, a small town (population 20,000) within 30 miles of a mid-sized metropolitan community. The area is reasonably competitive in terms of health care, with one community hospital and six other nursing facilities within a 30 mile radius. The full range of long-term care services, from assisted living to dementia care units, is available.

Whispering Pines Nursing and Rehabilitation Center is owned by a medium-sized nursing home corporation, American Family Health Care (AFHC), which owns or manages 58 facilities, each with 100 to 250 beds (see corporate Organization Chart, Figure 5.1). A regional vice president for management operations and a corporate nurse consultant for care standards and training make assessment visits to WPNRC at least quarterly. All AFHC long-term care facilities have corporate resources available to them, which include: corporate nurse consultant (training and corporate care standards), regional nursing consultants (assigned group of homes), corporate field accountant (business operations), marketing director, registered dietician, and regional vice president (facility management).

Figure 5.1 American Family Health Care Organization Chart

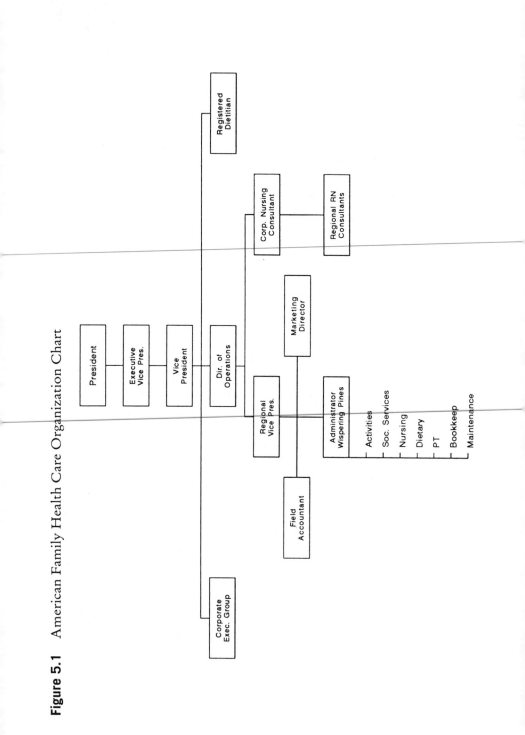

The corporation maintains oversight of all its facilities through its director of operations. Quarterly corporate reviews focus almost entirely on the fiduciary details—profit and loss statements, census figures, and labor costs. Only with the corporatewide initiative in Total Quality Management (TQM) have quarterly reviews begun to focus more on reductions in variability of resident care outcomes from the quality of operations.

The current administrator of WPNRC, Mary Rose, has managed the facility for five years. The corporation, however, has owned the facility for only three years. Mary Rose grew up in Tarleton Springs and comes from a well-respected family with deep roots in the community. She has over 20 years of long-term care management experience.

Whispering Pines' director of nursing (DON), Alice Masters, has nearly 30 years of nursing experience, almost all of it in acute care settings. Masters was hired as the DON one year ago. She came to Whispering Pines on short notice when the previous director resigned suddenly. Her selection was based on weak competition among applicants for the job, her strong management skills, and the perceived weakness in "people skills" possessed by the assistant director of nursing (ADON), Virginia Peeler. Peeler resigned in protest the day Masters was hired.

Nursing aides turn over frequently at Whispering Pines, since opportunities for aides are quite good locally. Competitors are paying aides between $1 and $1.50 per hour more than WPNRC. Despite Rose's reputation for managing effectively, she has not reduced nursing aide turnover rates. Before the TQM program was implemented, these rates exceeded 100 percent annually. That was one reason Rose requested that Whispering Pines be one of the first six corporate facilities to implement TQM.

The range of care given at WPNRC includes traditional nursing home care, subacute care (20 beds), and Alzheimer's care (10 beds). Restorative programs are active in dining, incontinence management, progressive mobility, physical restraint use, and cognitive orientation. Rose believes that aide turnover rates and weak management by the former director and assistant director of nursing have inhibited solid, restorative program development.

The corporate nurse consultant, Ms. Joan Morgan, worked with the administrator and department heads to start the TQM project. It included a TQM Steering Committee composed of the directors of social services, nursing, activities, dietetics, physical therapy, assistant director of nursing, and the business office manager, with Rose ex officio. The TQM program they developed focused on resident restorative care activities. Ms. Morgan spent four days in the facility helping the DON teach and begin TQM concepts with staff on all shifts.

Ed Taggert, corporate regional vice president, oversees WPNRC and 11 other facilities. During his most recent visit two months ago, Taggert told Rose that if the restorative programs did not start showing significant improvement by his June visit, her bonus would be in jeopardy. Moreover, corporate would likely increase its role in determining the mix of residents admitted to WPNRC.

Rounds I

Rose was walking her rounds with Alice Masters when Lizy Jones came up to them rapidly. With tears rolling down her cheeks she asked, "Why isn't it working, Ms. Rose? Why isn't it getting any better?"

"What is the matter Lizy? You need to slow down a bit and let Alice and me help you."

"Well, Ms. Rose, it's the TQM program. I've gone to all those meetings you had where you talked about improvement programs. You said the residents were going to get easier to take care of and their lives would be better. After three months the residents want just as much, and some of them don't want to even do their restorative programs."

"Come Lizy, it can't be all that bad. Mrs. Harriston's daughter was in just yesterday saying she was impressed that her mom had improved her mobility and was also eating more independently. Surely, Millie's gains under your assistance show that TQM is working."

"Mrs. Harriston has improved. I know from the care planning group I am on, as well as from her being one of my permanent assignments. But Mrs. Harriston still yells and hits at the nurses and aides as much as she ever did. She is just as mean to the other residents when she doesn't get as much attention as she wants. TQM classes were to help get our work done easier and faster if we did our part. But it hasn't made our shifts any easier."

"Oh come, Lizy," started Alice Masters, "we all know that a few teams being formed and a philosophy like TQM is not going to turn WPNRC into heaven in a couple of months. Give it time. Work with it."

"Why? The nurses aren't practicing it! Most of the aides, at least the ones I know, have been trying their best. We may not be perfect like you said we had to be, but we are doing the best we can with what we have to work with." Lizy turned and stormed back toward her work area.

Rose turned toward Masters. "Is she right Alice?" Alice replied with agitation, "The nurses have gone through the training but their hearts are not fully in it. It seemed so artificial. There is so much record keeping to do, besides providing care, that the idea of no errors is violated daily. With our wage scale, WPNRC is just a place to gain experience before they can work at one of the city's hospitals."

"Well, I have to know how well it is working out," Mary replied. "You better have an extra TQM staff meeting this week. If things are not working, we have to fix them up before Taggert's scheduled June corporate visit. Give me a complete assessment report in two weeks. If you need some help, call Joan Morgan, the nurse consultant who provided our training in TQM at corporate."

Weekly Nursing Department Meeting

Alice began, "Let's look at the restorative programs on Two East. We should be having at least a 20 percent increased success rate in the dining program and 15 percent in the progressive mobility program. What do you have for the wing, Diane?"

Diane Wells, the assistant director of nursing, began slowly. "Well, Alice, while the average for the residents in the entire facility fits our average planned gains, there are very significant variances. Also, there are important regressions for some residents. Two East, specifically, has not achieved even half of their targeted outcome goals.

"I think it has a lot to do with Lizy Jones and her friends, especially Clara Smith and Paula Whitson. They were weak in the training classes. When they got out on the floor they returned to their old ways, like so many other aides."

"I am not sure Diane. Just two days ago Ms. Rose and I had Lizy come up to us in tears. She was challenging the nursing staff to get on board. Lizy seemed very upset that TQM was not working."

"Well, I don't know about other sections of the home, but I personally know all the staff nurses that serve on Two East. Those nurses are some of the finest nurses in the facility."

Alice could feel tension rising as she said, "I am not one to support an aide over nurses, but we must make this TQM thing work better. Ms. Rose was quite clear with me. I can't go to her and say that petty bickering between staff levels is causing TQM not to work. We have to stop personalizing everything and think more in terms of outcomes, processes, and systems. Use the care planning sessions in the next two weeks to see that nursing acts as a team with dietary, activities, and social work."

Diane was feeling pressured to answer more enthusiastically regarding the TQM project, "Okay, Alice, but meetings won't cure what ails us. It's salaries and work conditions. We need higher salaries. We need more staff. More TQM will not be enough. After all, we are professionals and we always do our professional best."

Alice made a mental note to work on the nursing aide team observations record keeping. "Okay, let's move on to the quality assurance report. We've talked enough about TQM. By the way, there is a joint TQM meeting of all of our regional homes at corporate headquarters. Does anyone want to volunteer to go?" The meeting room fell silent for a long time.

"Well, there may be more people than Lizy Jones having trouble TQ-ing in this facility. Let's have it all—the good and the ugly." The room was filled with noise and highly charged emotions for the next 30 minutes.

When Alice Masters closed her office door, she felt a headache coming on. She could sense that she was going to have her work cut out for her in completing Ms. Rose's report. Alice was used to organizing, but only within the context of hospital operations where hierarchies were clear and delegation could be depended upon. Alice had a strong record of fostering teamwork among self-motivated professionals. Unfortunately for Alice, TQM compressed hierarchies, replacing them with process improvement teams run by those closest to the problems and needs of customers. She really didn't know how one would communicate the tenets of TQM to aides and nurses.

Alice thought awhile, then summarized on her note pad, the positive elements of the TQM activities she had discovered during the first five months of its implementation:

- Five TQM restorative programs were operational, including dining, progressive mobility, physical restraint reduction, cognitive orientation, and incontinence management.
- Dining restorative programs increased independent eating by 21 percent, consistent with care plans.
- Progressive mobility program gains were on schedule for the predicted 15 percent improvement within one year of adaption of TQM.
- Ten percent fewer residents needed physical restraints for their personal safety.
- Family surveys indicating service excellence for the facility were up 30 percent in the quality of life areas, and had moved from 61 percent to 78 percent for nursing care areas.
- Pearson Memorial, locally, and the two hospitals in the city were referring 11 percent more subacute care resident candidates to WPNRC compared to the year before.

While the positive effects, or seemingly positive effects, of the TQM program were impressive, the negatives she would have to report to Ms. Rose were disturbing, and perhaps even disastrous if Alice knew Taggert and corporate central. The main negative results of the TQM program included the following:

- Certified nursing aide turnover was at a three-year high, reaching 125 percent on an annual basis.
- The assistant director of nursing was not committed to TQM.
- Two East had a negative influence on total facility results by at least 15 percent.
- Following four training sessions given over a two-week period by the corporate nursing consultant, nearly half of the nursing staff did not understand or practice TQM. During her rounds and her review of the paperwork, Alice saw little evidence of data-driven problem solving in resident care, nurse assistant empowerment, or adequate continuing training.
- Salaries in the facility were lagging, falling almost $.60 per hour behind other service opportunities in town and a full $1.50 behind overall opportunities in the city.
- Blaming fellow staff for care lapses, as opposed to searching for system problems, had not diminished.
- TQM seemed to be working best with the easiest residents to improve and the best nursing aides; therefore, the statistical gains in resident quality of life and quality of care were overstated.
- Ms. Rose was being criticized as being unrealistic for having launched five restorative programs at once.

Rounds II

The report Rose had requested from Alice Masters on TQM progress and the problems on Two East was now two weeks late. Taggert's scheduled visit was only a month away. The TQM program was in its fifth month after training (see Table 5.1, implementation schedule). What had started out so positively with corporate training eight months ago, followed with training for all staff by Jane Morgan, corporate nurse consultant, had become derailed. Somehow the hopefulness of quality enhancements for residents had turned into a personnel and overall facility nightmare for Rose.

Rose stared out at the parking lot. The most recent month's certified nursing aide (CNA) turnover rate had gone above the historical monthly rate for the first time since the TQM program started. The rate was now clearly above corporate standards. The morning review of census statistics showed a decline, and Two East was becoming a census problem of the first proportion. Only the continuing strong financial showing of the fully occupied subacute care and Alzheimer's units were keeping the facility in the black.

Rose was thankful that she had hired Alice a year ago, since she was providing such strong leadership to the subacute area. She was also glad

Table 5.1   TQM Implementation at Whispering Pines: Year One

Facilitywide training by corporate nurse consultant	Mid-September
Follow-up training by director of nursing and clinical nurse coordinator	Late September
Full program implementation/team formation	Mid-December
Regional vice president visit	Early March
Nurse aide outburst on TQM program	Late March
Special department meeting on TQM	Early April
DON assessment of TQM report due	April 15
Early visit of regional vice president	Early May
Fire assistant director of nursing	Mid-May
Regional vice president visit	June 10
Resignation of DON	June 17
Regional vice president visit	August 15

that Alice had suggested a pay differential ladder for nurses working the subacute area. The subacute area's low turnover rate was a thing to be proud of. On the other hand, only the dining and mobility programs in the restorative areas had proven to be successful under TQM. In fact, facility-wide incontinence was on the rise, and Activities had been reporting a significant decline in attendance and socialization in facility-sponsored social activities for the past three months.

Rose left her office to begin her daily rounds. She knew that Alice was likely to be on Two East due to the change of the shifts at 3 p.m. Alice would be listening to the floor report, since the floor had been defined as a "facility must-watch area" over the last four weeks. Rose got off the elevator and went directly to where Masters was leading the month-end TQ shift change mini-session on quality of life and care for the wing.

"Alice, I really need to talk with you about your progress on the TQM report right after this session."

"Well, we might as well do it now then," Alice replied. "I only have three more residents' restorative programs to discuss. The rest of the shift change can be covered by Eileen. Okay, Eileen?"

"Sure, Alice, I have all the necessary records and documentation right here. You and I discussed these cases yesterday. Also, I need to cover some lapses with the aides regarding care plans, especially Lizy Jones."

Rose's Office

Alice Masters quietly closed the door. She began, "I'm sorry the report is two weeks late, but it's taken far longer than I thought it would."

"I really do appreciate your concern, Alice, but I guess it's time for the truth—the whole truth. Don't hold anything back today."

"It's really not pretty, and I am a little disappointed in myself for not staying on top of it. The bottom line is, unfortunately, close to Taggert's early-on assessment from when you and he had the meeting shortly before TQM was implemented. I think Taggert was unhappy that corporate sided with you and subsidized the training as one of six corporate pilots."

Masters' assessment was that TQM was progressively losing impact. In fact, it was breaking down and breaking apart. From her observations, interviews with key staff, review of family surveys, regular TQM planning sessions, and regular facility meetings, she was able to assess the TQM effort more fully. The facility still lacked a quality rewards and recognition program. Permanently assigned key nursing aides, informal leaders, several shift nurses, and the ADON definitely were not TQM advocates. This large group had never accepted the concepts of teamwork and continuous improvement. They preferred and strongly believed in quality assurance systems and hierarchial controls with a basic task process orientation toward resident services and care.

Also, the record keeping for the facility for the subacute care unit and the Minimum Data Set cut dramatically into the data development necessary for the TQM process. While most permanently assigned nursing aides accepted and practiced TQM in its basic aspects, residents encountered enough nurses and nursing aides, particularly on weekends, that didn't lead them to lose respect for the program. While dietary was a strong practitioner of TQM concepts and approaches to problem solving, including requirements for continual training, this was not common in other support areas. Activities and social work were less than enthusiastic in their support, and were very inconsistent in their practice.

Masters continued her report by discussing the facilitywide TQM Steering Group, which had canceled, delayed, or run incomplete meetings during three of the five months of its existence due to competing work schedules and unplanned resident care interruptions. Masters noted that she would be happy to do TQM if she could. However, the TQM program at Whispering Pines was not suited to her. It didn't fit her hospital training, and her personality was far more directive than the TQM philosophy required.

Masters ended her assessment of the six months of TQM at Whispering Pines by noting that Rose herself had not followed through with daily role modeling on her facility rounds. There was frequent discussion that she did not "walk the talk," but reprimanded and instructed during the rounds in the same fashion as she did before TQM. Also, she kept decisions and information almost entirely to herself. For example, the key decision on how many restorative programs to implement at one time was hers, and was not discussed thoroughly with nursing, to say nothing of the permanently assigned aides. Another example of decision making without adequate sharing was the decision to accelerate subacute care, TQM, and restorative programs without any planned and communicated phase-in schedule. Finally, everyone awaited her promised rewards and recognition program that was supposed to have been a visible, high-quality program. The actual program, however, consisted of a certificate and a meal, and was very similar to the old "Employee of the Month" designation.

When Masters finished her report, Rose questioned why she had not given her some assessment earlier. And why did she leave the ADON relatively unsupervised and in charge at critical points of the implementation process?

Alice flushed and said, "I guess I thought it might work out anyway. Also, I really thought you knew and didn't want to hear the negatives since they were so obvious."

"Do you have any idea how we can repair it, even if I have to take significant heat from Taggert and corporate? I know that TQM is the wave of the future for health care, including long-term care. Whether or not our employees are talented or ready, they can grow into it. Really, deep down, I know we've made some start-up mistakes, perhaps overextended ourselves, but that's all reversible if we just implement the right strategy. So what do you recommend? How can we get it back on track?"

Alice hesitated and looked down at the floor.

"Come on," continued Rose. "Deming always said that 80 to 85 percent of all problems in organizations are system problems and problems traceable to systematic variation, not people problems and random or specific variation. Why should we be different? Maybe we should fire a few employees. But really, we must have taken the wrong track somewhere in the implementation and training process. Let's try again. The residents' quality of life depends on it! I've been in this business for over twenty years and this is an idea whose time has come. Corporate was behind me. Alice, you just have to help me make it work. Use some of your strong management and supervision skills and make it happen. I know you can."

Westmount Nursing Homes, Incorporated: Implementing a Continuous Quality Improvement Initiative

Kent V. Rondeau

SHIRLEY CARPENTER took a deep breath and looked at her watch. It was 3:40 p.m. and there was just 20 minutes left to get ready for her 4 p.m. meeting with the board. She knew there was going to be a difficult confrontation, and believed that many board members would call into question her leadership skills and administrative judgement. She felt that her well-earned reputation as a brilliant strategist and dynamic change agent would be put to a severe test. She needed to find a way to calm the widespread fear that the total quality management (TQM) initiative she had worked so hard to implement at Westmount Nursing Homes was badly off the rails. She wondered what had gone wrong, and how it could be saved.

Background

Shirley Carpenter came to Westmount 22 months ago to assume the role of president and chief executive officer. Westmount Nursing Homes Incorporated is a for-profit chain of seven nursing homes located in a northeastern state. Since 1953, it had grown from a single 42-bed residential facility for affluent seniors to a dynamic company comprised

While the events in this case are based on actual nursing facility experiences, the names of the organization and of individuals represented have been changed to assure anonymity.

of four divisions: (1) the Facilities Division, managing skilled nursing homes; (2) the Home Care Division, operating homemaker and nursing services for seniors in their own homes; (3) the commissary services division, operating a central kitchen preparing and distributing meals to four of its homes, two small local hospitals, and elderly persons in their own homes; and (4) the consulting division, marketing management consulting and accounting services to a variety of clients in the long-term care industry. Westmount's statement of profit and loss for the past three years can be found in Table 6.1.

Westmount continues to search vigorously for opportunities to expand its core business. Last year it began a comprehensive day care program for seniors at five of its homes. Recently, discussions have been undertaken with Breton Funeral Homes to purchase its assets, including four family-owned funeral establishments. Westmount has also commenced negotiations with a regional chain of drug stores to lease them commercial space in its three largest homes. It also is exploring establishing a home care alliance with two other hospital-based home care programs in order to attract new managed care contracts and to improve referrals from existing contracts involving their parent hospitals.

Table 6.1 Westmount Nursing Homes Incorporated Statement of Revenue and Expenses (199x–199z) (figures in thousands of dollars)

	199x	199y	199z
Facilities Division			
Revenue	15,640	18,622	26,453
Expenses	12,458	15,140	22,512
Profit margin (%)	20.3	18.7	14.9
Home Care Division			
Revenue	1,741	2,254	3,060
Expenses	1,360	1,752	2,493
Profit margin (%)	21.9	22.3	18.5
Commissary Services Division			
Revenue	1,382	1,940	2,188
Expenses	1,263	1,614	1,870
Profit margin (%)	15.9	16.8	14.5
Consulting Division			
Revenue	—	42	426
Expenses	—	16	230
Profit margin (%)	—	61.9	46.0

Over the past three years, under the leadership of Shirley Carpenter, Westmount purchased two additional nursing homes, increasing its total skilled nursing bed complement by almost 43 percent. A strategic planning process was begun last year. Out of this initiative came Westmount's formal declaration to pursue the goal of becoming the "home of choice" in the tri-state area. Its primary target market was identified as affluent seniors who desire a broad range of single access, high-quality health and social services. This strategy was based on the belief that to survive in a rapidly changing health care environment, customers require "one stop shopping" for a wide variety of services outside of the acute care setting. Westmount firmly believes that future success will go to those proactive organizations which achieve a vertically and horizontally integrated delivery system.

Shirley Carpenter

Shirley Carpenter, RN, MBA, came to Westmount Nursing Homes two years ago from Grasslands Community General Hospital, where she had been the vice president of nursing. Grasslands is a 325-bed acute care hospital located in a rapidly growing community in the Midwest. At Grasslands, Shirley was widely received as a dynamic and resourceful leader who was not afraid of making the difficult decisions that went with her job description. She was primarily responsible for Grasslands' radical redesign of its patient care delivery system towards a highly integrated patient-focused approach. The changes she had initiated saved the hospital more than $1.7 million a year on direct patient care services, while at the same time lowered hospital length of stay and improved patient outcomes. When the press got wind of Grasslands' successful reorganization, the hospital and Shirley received a great deal of local and national media attention. Grasslands became recognized as an innovative organization at the cutting edge of excellence in patient care delivery. It wasn't long before Shirley was being asked to speak at forums about a wide variety of health care issues. She also received additional recognition when she was selected as "one of the most outstanding young health care executives in the nation."

Although the changes Shirley had instituted were widely acclaimed as successful, she did have her detractors. Her direct, no-nonsense style was often seen as confrontational, and many found her to be intellectually intimidating. On several occasions she had openly chastised staff members with whom she took issue. Although she was greatly respected and even admired by her staff, people tended to give her a wide berth on most issues. Shirley demanded perfection from her staff but also held herself up to the very highest level of performance expectation. She once stated, "You've got to be visible and out front if you're are going to navigate an organization toward progressive change. This requires that you stand behind your words and accept the consequences of your convictions. Complacency never got the job done. Too many people are attached to the status quo. You can't make an omelette without breaking a few eggs."

George Pearson had been the chief executive officer at Grasslands during Shirley Carpenter's tenure. George once stated that Shirley was "the daughter I never had." He had given her wide latitude and regularly deferred to her judgement in most areas related to running the hospital. Everyone had assumed that George had been grooming Shirley to take over the hospital upon his pending retirement. When he departed, the selection committee did the unexpected and chose another candidate. Shirley was devastated; six weeks later, she left Grasslands for Westmount Nursing Homes.

A New Direction for Westmount

Shirley Carpenter's arrival at Westmount created a great deal of anticipation and excitement. Her reputation as a health care innovator and progressive change agent was now well-established. Westmount had languished through a series of rather bland administrators over the years who lacked the vision that could move the organization forcefully into the twenty-first century.

The first year of Shirley's tenure at Westmount was marked by a number of bold initiatives on her part. Soon after arriving, she was able to dissipate the threat of loss of licensure and potential funding on two of its nursing homes that had been cited for a number of violations. Shirley also instituted a broad and sweeping reorganization at Westmount in creating the four operating divisions. In addition, after securing support from her board, Shirley began a very aggressive program of asset diversification because the firm had relied for too long on revenues from its affiliate homes. Declining reimbursement rates, coupled with full occupancy, meant that Westmount needed to broaden its base of revenue. This was partially achieved by expansion of its home care and food commissary services, and by establishing a consulting division to market management services to a variety of clients in the long-term care industry. In particular, the Consulting Division was thought to have significant growth potential due to a perceived lack of expertise by most local consultants on long-term care management issues. During this period, Westmount also purchased two additional homes with the option of acquiring three more. The firm spent more than $1.5 million on renovations to these facilities.

Within 18 months, Shirley had implemented a number of innovative programs at Westmount focused on providing augmented services to its seniors, and, in addition, began to expanded employee services. Shirley formed and chaired a quality of work life committee aimed at improving conditions for Westmount's employees and staff. Morale in all of the homes had suffered after years of neglect. At the time of Shirley's arrival, the turnover level of staff nurses and nursing assistants at Westmount was among the highest in the state. To reverse this, a recognition and performance based pay system was implemented identifing and rewarding outstanding individual and group achievement. A career planning and inventory program was developed to assist employees in identifying their career goals and charting a path toward these goals. In addition, the staff education and development program was greatly expanded. All employees were openly encouraged and received financial support to acquire their high school equivalency or to seek further education and skills enhancement. Westmount also established a progressive literacy program to address the intractable problem of illiteracy in the work place. The quality of work life committee estimated that about 35 percent of the workforce at Westmount had deficiencies in reading and writing. Shirley once stated that "organizational excellence comes about only when people are sufficiently motivated and empowered to make a difference. The bedrock of staff empowerment is knowledge and education. This requires a significant investment in the intellectual potential of each employee. Our people are our most important asset."

The Total Quality Management Initiative

Three months after arriving at Westmount, Shirley initiated a strategic planning retreat to identify Westmount's preferred future. One conclusion emerging from the retreat was that there was a need to find a way to better address quality of care issues in delivering services to seniors. Shirley latched on to the notion that total quality management (TQM) would be the vehicle through which Westmount could achieve the cultural transformation articulated in its vision statement, which included a statement that "Westmount Nursing Homes, Incorporated believes in striving for excellence in everything we do."

Shirley quickly became immersed in the burgeoning literature on total quality management. Her interest in and passion for its possibilities grew. In fact, she was so determined to become an expert in its theory and application that she began to explore the possibility of focusing her doctoral dissertation in this area.

Her faculty advisor and mentor was Dr. Daylon Quinby, a sage yet crusty academic, now nearing retirement. Shirley asked the venerable professor if he would "lead the quality improvement journey at Westmount." Dr. Quinby readily agreed, and was soon found wandering around the grounds at all hours observing people at work or showing up quite unannounced at management committee meetings. Several staff members found Dr. Quinby to be "an odd old duck" whose presence was somewhat annoying, if not unnerving. Most people did not know why he was there; some speculated that it was management's way of spying on them.

One of Dr. Quinby's first activities was to evaluate the organizational culture in the seven nursing homes. Findings from the cultural audit, used to assess readiness to pursue organizational change, indicated that much work would be required to transform Westmount. In particular, the professor found that prevailing work practices at Westmount were, in many respects, antithetical to the philosophy of TQM. Dr. Quinby announced the findings of the cultural audit at the semiannual general meeting of board, management, and staff. He stated in his address that "if Westmount is to successfully implement total quality management, no less than a total and unequivocable repudiation of current work place values and norms needs to be achieved." Quinby further stated that "the management in the homes consistently demonstrates patterns of practice that are overly autocratic, rigid, and dysfunctional. All too often, management treats its employees like little children. Employees respond by behaving as if management believes they can't be trusted. An overly confrontational atmosphere, based on suspicion bordering on paranoia, has created an element of fear surrounding and pervading work in many of the homes." Dr. Quinby cited several examples from incidents he had observed. Needless to say, the conclusions he rendered were not well-received by a number of members of the staff and managers.

Soon after the cultural audit feedback sessions, Shirley Carpenter and 12 senior managers embarked on a ten-day educational retreat to learn the tools and techniques of TQM and the leadership skills needed to successfully navigate the cultural transformation it required. Although the retreat was located on a resort island in the Caribbean, Shirley impressed on her managers that the time spent was not a paid holiday, but an opportunity to acquire new leadership and management skills. When the news broke that management had gone to a resort for a "working retreat," many employees openly questioned why they needed to "go so far away to learn how to manage better at home."

When the senior managers returned from the retreat, many could scarcely contain their enthusiasm, and set about immediately to apply the principles they had learned. A quality council was quickly formed, chaired jointly by Shirley Carpenter and Dr. Quinby. The quality council was charged with leading and directing the TQM transformation at Westmount. Its membership consisted of the directors of the seven homes and the divisional directors of home care, commissary services, and consulting services, along with senior representatives from human resources and strategic planning. Within two weeks, executives in each of the homes and divisions were busy holding educational seminars for their middle managers and supervisors on the philosophy, tools, and techniques of TQM.

It wasn't long afterward, under the supervision by the quality council, that the first quality improvement (QI) team was formed. Led by Shirley Carpenter and facilitated by Dr. Quinby, a seven-member multifunctional team of service providers suggested innovative ways to dramatically reduce the waiting period for nursing response to requests from bedridden residents. Within two months, 23 QI teams examined quality related problems ranging from improving resident food to designing a new commercial exercise video program for seniors. Table 6.2 provides a list of these early quality improvement projects at Westmount.

Initial interest and excitement generated by many employees for the TQM initiative at Westmount convinced Shirley that she was on to something big. Many of her junior managers, however, were privately expressing fear that the changes, which now were transforming Westmount's once placid culture, were happening all too fast. Vice president of Finance Norm Taylor's opinion was shared by many other managers at Westmount: "It's a proven fact that people in the long-term care industry really can't absorb organizational change as easily as those working in acute care settings. People here just have too much respect for tradition and past practice."

For her part, Shirley was strongly convinced that these changes could not occur fast enough. Shirley stated, "I don't believe in waiting around and hoping that something good comes your way. That just never happens. I like to create success right away. One small victory produces another, and soon you've won the war. The fact is, people like to associate with winners."

The Westmount Board Responds

The board of Westmount was never really very enthusiastic about Shirley's TQM makeover. Explained to them as a tool to enhance productivity

Table 6.2 Westmount Nursing Homes Incorporated Quality
Improvement Projects

QI Program	Responsibility
1. Client satisfaction survey	Headquarters
2. Family satisfaction survey	Headquarters
3. Nursing response times	Facilities
4. Seniors' exercise video	Headquarters
5. Staff retention study	Facilities
6. Guest relations study	Headquarters
7. Medication errors	Facilities
8. Suggestion system design	Headquarters
9. Resident fall study	Facilities
10. Wandering patients study	Facilities
11. Employee recognition program	Headquarters
12. Patient accounts	Headquarters
13. Food quality	Facilities
14. Food preparation	Headquarters
15. Pet therapy	Headquarters
16. Job redesign	Headquarters
17. Physician reimbursement	Headquarters
18. Physician satisfaction	Headquarters
19. Ethical review	Facilities
20. Grounds beautification	Facilities
21. Resident transportation	Facilities
22. Self-scheduling	Facilities
23. New Ventures	Headquarters

and create a long-term competitive advantage in Westmount's chosen
markets, the board reluctantly gave its approval "to implement a TQM
program, as long as it wasn't too costly." The chairperson of the board
was Dr. Ann Howard, age 57, a highly respected family physician with
a specialty in geriatric medicine who was a long-time board member.
Dr. Howard was not convinced that TQM could work at Westmount,
and stated, "Total quality management might be all right for building
cars, but I just can't understand how it can work in a nursing home.
Anyway, I read somewhere that this TQM stuff is just an expensive fad,
and that over 80 percent of health care organizations who have tried to
implement it have failed. Can we really afford to try something with such
a spotty track record? Perhaps Shirley should be spending her time and
the organization's money on proven management methods."

Shirley knew that the turnaround at Westmount would not happen
overnight. She chalked up the board's indifference to ignorance, and
resolved that she would not be deterred from her quest to transform

Westmount. "Give me three years and you won't recognize this place," she was heard to have said.

Labor Contract Negotiations Begin

Several months after the TQM initiative had begun, Westmount began contract negotiations with the local chapter of the United Federation of Nurses, representing Westmount's 214 registered nurses and nurse assistants. Shirley believed in taking a hands-on approach to dealing with the unions, and insisted on conducting all negotiations personally. In the beginning, management at Westmount felt that contract discussions would be straightforward and would proceed with little of the rancor that had characterized much of their collective bargaining in the past. In the earliest months of the TQM initiative, Westmount had witnessed a remarkable improvement in work place morale. It was hoped that improved morale would pay an important "peace dividend" with the organization, winning important concessions from the union.

In fact, all three of the unions representing nonmanagement employees at Westmount believed that the active participation of their membership in TQM demonstrated their steadfast commitment to finding new ways of working responsibly with management. For many years, the fractious nature of their contract negotiations had left both sides bitter after they had concluded.

From the union's vantage point, negotiations were aimed at improving the collective agreement by obtaining significant wage gains and achieving formal union representation on the Westmount board. Two issues were of particular significance during contract talks. First, the union sought to replace the merit pay plan for registered nurses with an across-the-board pay increase for all nurses. Most people felt the merit pay plan, conceived to reward top performers, was not working very well. Many viewed it as a complicated and subjective protocol that caused a great deal of confusion and bitterness in its application. Second, the union sought protection against what they felt was management's abhorrent practice of substituting RNs with certified nursing assistants (CNAs) and other personal care workers. The union claimed that management was using lower paid nursing auxiliaries for tasks which legally should be done by RNs.

Early in the contract negotiations it became apparent that they would be very difficult indeed. In its opening address at the negotiation table, the union stated that its "price of compliance" with Westmount's total quality program was significant wage increases for its membership. Shirley countered by offering to provide job security and suggesting to form a committee to study questions of nursing labor deployment. She also stated that she was in favor of allowing union representation on the board. This was consistent with her idea of incorporating more vibrant forms of employee participation in the work place. However, Shirley insisted that the merit pay plan must remain in place. As its architect, she felt a deep personal commitment to its consumation. Shirley stated, "You've got to have a way of rewarding those people who consistently perform above the call of duty. That's what quality service is all about. Pay is a great way to motivate people. To ignore the impact money has on the performance of employees is to remove a very powerful weapon from your arsenal." After several heated meetings, the negotiations seemed to be at an impasse.

The Board Steps In

It was soon apparent to the Westmount board that contract negotiations with the nurse's union were not going well. The executive committee of the board met with Shirley to determine an appropriate strategy to help an agreement be reached. After much heated discussion, they decided that management should take a more direct approach in dealing with the union. Dr. Howard summed up the attitude of the board in saying that, "You can't allow a union to ruin the financial viability of your enterprise. The truth is, eighty percent of our costs are direct expenditures for labor. If we are ever to reverse our fiscal problems around here, we need to get control of our labor costs. These people have to realize we're all in this thing together." The board also gave a thumb's down to the idea of allowing union representation on the board. Dr. Howard remarked, "You know, this move to democratize the work place is just a bunch of rampant socialism. You give these people an inch and they take a mile."

When Shirley returned to the bargaining table, she brought along Dr. Quinby to assist in discussions. Unfortunately, he was not able to expedite breaking the impasse. His abrasive and abrupt manner further alienated the union and created additional tensions at the table. With no new offer made by either side, no resolution on any of the major outstanding issues could be achieved. Shirley suspended negotiations by claiming that the union was being inflexible while "holding the residents of the homes ransom for a few extra pennies."

The Flash Point

At this point the executive committee of the board began to make direct overtures to union representatives requesting an informal meeting to "determine if there were not avenues of mutual interest that could be

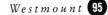

explored." Dr. Howard and two other board members met in private with the union negotiators and suggested the possibility of major staff cuts if the union did not agree to make significant wage concessions. The union representatives countered by insinuating that the Westmount management was bargaining in bad faith. Robert Sawyer, the chief negotiator, said, "We will not be bullied into signing a collective agreement that does not have the best interests of our membership at heart. We have showed our willingness to bargain in good conscience by engaging in activities aimed at improving productivity. The participation of our members in these efforts is often unpaid and obviously unappreciated." The meeting ended with the union threatening to boycott further participation by its membership in future quality improvement activities. According to Robert Sawyer, "If we are going to be treated with such contempt, I can only recommend to my membership that we suspend our active participation in this program immediately."

As Shirley prepared for the 4 p.m. board meeting she was frustrated and angry that persons and events had conspired against her. She had always felt pride in her ability to control any agenda. Her record of achievement was one of soaring accomplishments. She wondered how she could regain control of her board and move ahead with the important reforms she had initiated.

Ethical Issues

Rockingham County Nursing Home: The Moral Dilemma of Creating an Institutional DNR Policy

Marc D. Hiller, James B. Lewis, and William F. Sturtevant

I: Is There a Problem?

Mrs. Ethel Quimby

ETHEL QUIMBY, 64 years of age, had been a resident of Rockingham County Nursing Home (RCNH) for two years. Following the death of her husband three years earlier, Mrs. Quimby vehemently resisted admission to a nursing facility in spite of her gradually deteriorating health. After months of persuasion, she finally agreed to admission to RCNH, based largely on the recommendation of her sister Lucille (who was the former mother-in-law of William Sturtevant, Administrator of RCNH) and of her daughter, Marjorie, who lived in Concord, New Hampshire, about 45 minutes west of the facility.

For the first year following admission Mrs. Quimby became moderately involved with the RCNH's extensive programs and formed friendships with one or two other residents. Marjorie was a frequent visitor. During these visits Mrs. Quimby continued to complain about her living situation; she wished to return home or to move in with Marjorie and her family.

This case is based on a real life situation that occurred at Rockingham County Nursing Home and that involved William F. Sturtevant, the facility's administrator. Other names have been fictionalized and information has been added to make the case more suitable for educational purposes. However, all critical facts, documents, and outcomes are real or true.

Gradually, Mrs. Quimby grew more dissatisfied with her environment and increasingly withdrawn. Her visits with Marjorie became confrontational and unpleasant. Marjorie sought advice from a variety of professionals, including RCNH staff, who suggested Mrs. Quimby be transferred to another county facility closer to Concord. Marjorie's transfer application was approved, and preparations were made.

On the day of the scheduled move Mrs. Quimby informed Marjorie and the RCNH staff that, after thinking it over, she had changed her mind and refused to move. Several days of unsuccessful cajoling followed, and Marjorie ultimately decided to leave her mother at RCNH.

Mrs. Quimby's depression deepened, and three weeks later she simply would not get out of bed. Several days of urging from Marjorie, RCNH staff, and clergy were unsuccessful. She was repeatedly informed of the health risks associated with her decision to remain immobile. Consultants evaluating her case believed Mrs. Quimby was refusing to leave her bed to punish Marjorie for placing her in a nursing facility in the first place and for not visiting her more often.

Within a few weeks, Mrs. Quimby developed breathing difficulties and she was transferred to a local community hospital for evaluation and treatment. Shortly after admission Mrs. Quimby developed severe pneumonia and was placed on a ventilator. She had not previously executed an advance directive. Her attending physician, Dr. Bridges from RCNH, did not support the hospital's decision, as he believed she would not be motivated to get off of the ventilator. Marjorie and the other family members wanted "everything done for Mrs. Quimby." Mrs. Quimby died three months after admission to the hospital.

Within one month of Mrs. Quimby's death, Dr. Bridges told Mr. Sturtevant that his patient never should have been transferred or received life support at the hospital. RCNH had no policy on providing or withholding cardiopulmonary resuscitation (CPR). In this case, it was the hospital's policies that had prevailed. Dr. Bridges was concerned that although in this situation a "do not resuscitate" (DNR) order had not been an issue, future cases might occur at RCNH. He urged the administrator to open the issue of DNR to discussion among facility staff, and to consider establishing a written institutional policy on the issue. Mr. Sturtevant was responsive and suggested that Dr. Bridges take the lead in organizing the effort. Recognizing that this issue extended well beyond the medical care of individual residents, he tapped you, Ms. Waters, as assistant administrator, to spearhead the management team's efforts on resolving this institutional dilemma.

Dr. Bridges just telephoned you to schedule an initial meeting in two weeks to plan strategy. Taking out a legal pad, you begin to jot down preliminary ideas on how to proceed prior to and after your meeting with Dr. Bridges. On reflection, your notes distill to the following questions: Does RCNH even need a formal written institutional DNR policy? (Much can be said for not having anything down in writing.) Whom should we consult in determining whether there is a true need for such a policy? Whom should we consult in defining the elements of such a written policy? Who would be affected by this decision, and in what ways? What information do we need to arrive at a decision? What are the specific sources of this information? What are the key issues and considerations surrounding this written policy? Following a brief lunch, you return to your desk to tackle your list of questions.

Overview of Rockingham County Nursing Home

All New Hampshire counties own and operate at least one nursing home. Most of them have 100–150 beds; RCNH is among the largest with 300 intermediate care beds. The facility runs at a 99 percent occupancy rate, with a waiting list of 10 to 12 persons. Two-thirds of its residents are female. As a county facility, a large majority (93–95 percent) of RCNH residents are dependent on Medicaid, with few privately paying residents. The average age of residents is 84; the average length of stay is slightly over 36 months. RCNH's racial mix reflects the state's homogeneity, averaging between 1 and 3 percent minority residents.

The facility provides a higher level of care than most other intermediate care facilities (ICFs) around the state because of a high degree of dependency among its residents. The majority of RCNH residents are wheelchair bound or chair or bedfast. Fewer than one-third ambulate independently, and most require assistance in eating. All, except for one, require help in bathing. Having a significant number of residents suffering from dementia, it views itself as a special care "facility," as opposed to designating special care "units."

Market Position and Image

In many respects RCNH serves a unique market niche. Individuals not accepted by other facilities are admitted to RCNH; it is the nursing facility of last resort for residents of the county. According to its mission statement, RCNH "is committed to providing holistic care to its residents. The physical, emotional, spiritual, and psychological needs are addressed by qualified medical, nursing, and supportive allied health professionals. A safe, comfortable, home-like environment influenced by individual needs and preferences is provided with careful recognition of each resident's rights regarding confidentiality, safety, spirituality, and quality of life. A comprehensive team approach in providing care is directed according to achieving and maintaining the maximum potential of each resident." Many residents have intense medical needs, requiring heavy care, and some have extensive behavior problems, as well. In order to diversify its payer mix, the facility has targeted lighter care and private pay residents, bringing RCNH in direct competition with other area providers.

II: Developing a Formal DNR Policy

"Dr. Bridges to see you, Ms. Waters."

For the past two weeks, you have been preparing for this meeting with Dr. Bridges to discuss the desirability and appropriateness of developing an institutional DNR policy for RCNH. You know that Dr. Bridges will be well-prepared for the meeting. The idea of not having a written DNR policy initially appeared quite attractive to you. The facility had been in operation for decades and no problem had ever arisen because of a lack of written policy. The current situation was precipitated by care at the local hospital. Should Mrs. Quimby have been transferred to the hospital in the first place? That decision had been made according to current policy by the nursing supervisor on duty. Her decision was based on standing orders to transfer residents experiencing respiratory distress when a member of the medical staff cannot be contacted immediately. If the transfer had not been made and she had arrested at RCNH, it is unclear whether she would have been ventilated or whether CPR would have been initiated in the absence of institutional policies on these issues.

Upon further research you have become convinced that a written policy is advisable to avoid potential litigation and to create greater clarity for staff. In addition, Mr. Sturtevant is interested in settling this issue and feels it might require a written policy statement. In your opinion, creating such a policy requires extensive input from many individuals including physicians, nurses, and other caregivers, members of the management team, legal counsel, and potentially residents and their families. The final policy would have to be approved by the Board of Commissioners, so their input would be desirable as well. Given the public nature of RCNH, meetings on this issue would be open to the community and the media.

"Hello Clare. It looks like we've got a hot one here." Dr. Bridges came in and sat down at the conference table.

"I think you're right about that, Bob." You and Dr. Bridges both came to work at RCNH about the same time and you have an excellent professional relationship. Dr. Bridges began shuffling through a large stack of papers he brought in with him. "What is all that stuff, Bob?"

"Clare, you know I've been a physician a long time—some days it seems too long. Anyway, I started thinking back through my years at Rockingham and all the years before that, and I couldn't remember when CPR ever helped any patient who was on their way out. Sure, you hear about cases like that, and certainly it happens sometimes in hospitals and on television, but I've never been a part of a successful resuscitation in a nursing home. So, I decided to check it out, and do a little research on the subject."

Dr. Bridges continued, "First of all, you'd be surprised how little has been reported on this subject. I finally found one good study that looks like it's on target for us. Take a look at this information (see Figure 7.1); the bottom line is that CPR doesn't help old people in places like Rockingham."

The information handed to you by Dr. Bridges was pretty convincing. Of course, this was only one study, and you know it's always a bit risky to develop policy, particularly one this important, based on a single study.

After giving you a minute to look at the information, Dr. Bridges continued, "And, to make it even dicier, we need to somehow make sure that our staff—maybe all of them—are Advanced Cardiac Life Support (ACLS) certified. If we don't, we are really hanging out there for a lawsuit. I can just see it now. We advertise CPR, a code comes in, and some new employee, waiting for certification, is the only one around. What a mess that would be."

"That's a good point, Bob. As it is now, our staff members are not required to be ACLS-certified. The last survey we did showed that only about 15 percent of them are. We could always require all employees to be certified; that might not be a bad idea, but it would cost a lot . . . and all I need is more paperwork to keep track of."

"There's also the matter of a witnessed arrest," added Dr. Bridges. "Unless someone actually witnesses the arrest we have no way of knowing when it took place. We may do CPR, bring the resident back, and end up with a resident destined to 'live' in a persistent vegetative state, possibly for years . . . in our facility. And we know the personal impact of this on the resident's family and on our staff."

"That's another good point," you add. "Who has to be around to certify the arrest? And what training do they need? Will we have to train all the food service workers and volunteers to recognize an arrest, make a judgement call, and maybe even initiate CPR? There are a lot of cans full of worms involved in this issue."

"As far as I can tell from my conversations with physicians and staff, there's no unanimity on this. Most of the physicians want a DNR policy in writing . . . but not all of them. And a lot of nurses want to keep things

Figure 7.1 Outcomes of CPR in a Long-Term Care Facility (April 1987–August 1990)

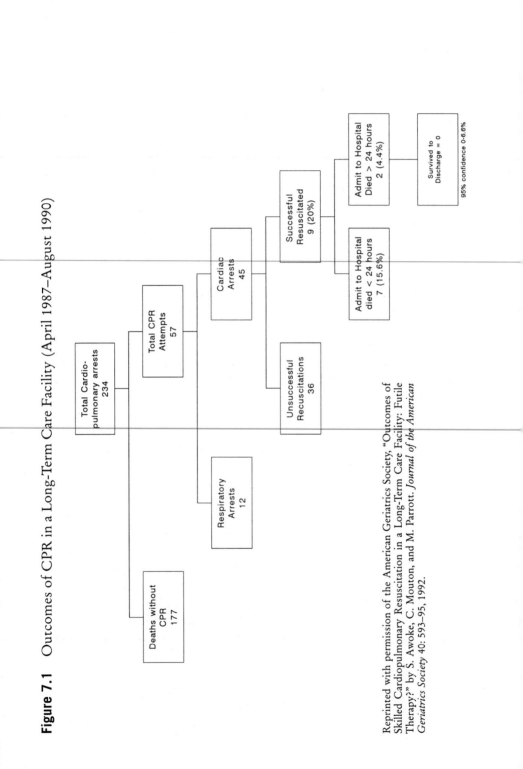

Reprinted with permission of the American Geriatrics Society, "Outcomes of Skilled Cardiopulmonary Resuscitation in a Long-Term Care Facility: Futile Therapy?" by S. Awoke, C. Mouton, and M. Parrott. *Journal of the American Geriatrics Society* 40: 593–95, 1992.

the way they are. I guess in a way that makes things easier for them on the floors. A couple of my best nurses said they're not sure they could work in a place that didn't at least try to resuscitate residents. Simply allowing residents to die without trying to save them violates what they view as their professional and moral obligation to sustain 'life' whenever possible. Some even feel this way for residents who have chosen to exercise their legal right to make an advance directive indicating they did not want to be resuscitated."

"Yes, I know. Dr. Beaudette is opposed to having a DNR policy," added Dr. Bridges. "A lot of us, not just here at Rockingham, are thinking that the courts and the public will take care of the problem for us. You know the new requirements on patient self-determination, living wills, and durable power of attorney for health care. They think the new requirements such as the Patient Self-Determination Act[1] will clear it up for us, but I'm not so sure. What do we do for the numerous residents who lack the capacity to request, or even to consent, to an advance directive? What about those who did, but who have since changed their minds, but not their original directive? What happens if the resident wants CPR, but we have a policy against it? Or even worse, what happens if the resident tells us that she does not want CPR attempted, goes into an arrest and loses consciousness, and the family demands that we 'just keep mom alive, no matter what.' I'm not sure how the courts would handle that one, but I can't imagine a facility going against the wishes of the family, whether there's a living will around or not."

"That's all true, Bob, but we have to move ahead on this. I've been talking with Bill Sturtevant and he agrees that we need to structure a group to wrestle with this one; you know I hate committees, but I don't know how we get around it here. I've put together a list of people I think ought to be involved. The way I see it, the group should be: Bill Sturtevant, all of the physicians, the director of nursing, the assistant director of nursing, the director of social services, the director of Pastoral Care, a geriatric nurse practitioner, and a staff nurse. What do you think?"

"Sounds a bit large, but you're probably on target; and you know, we have a couple other bases that should be touched, too. How about an attorney who can advise us of potential legal implications, and at least one of the county commissioners? They have to sign off on the whole thing anyway. What do you think about having residents and family members represented, and maybe even an ethicist who has experience in wrestling with this dilemma?"

You had been thinking about this issue, but had decided the size of the group was already large enough, so for now, at least, you were against the idea of its expansion. Dr. Bridges agreed to the limitation.

The first meeting of the ad hoc committee was convened two weeks later. News of the committee and the issue being discussed spread considerably during this time and you have been receiving numerous comments. Among the more interesting conversations you had was one with Marjorie, Mrs. Quimby's daughter, who wanted to make a presentation to the committee about her personal experience. After much discussion with Dr. Bridges, you agreed to invite Marjorie. Her presentation opens the meeting.

In her comments Marjorie strongly and emotionally expressed her view that resuscitation was not appropriate for her mother. "We thought at the time that everything should be done to keep her alive, that some miracle would take place to bring her back the way we knew her. We were wrong. Watching her hooked up like that was hell. If you ever have to be in that position again—and I imagine you will, please . . . think about the family, think about the resident; don't feel you have to play God. Please."

Following Marjorie, Dr. Bridges presented the results of his research showing the ineffectiveness of CPR, especially among the elderly, as well as the issues surrounding a witnessed arrest. Whereas Marjorie's presentation was received in silent respect, Dr. Bridges' comments sparked lively debate.

As had been anticipated, Dr. Beaudette strongly held that it was his moral responsibility to do everything he possibly could to prolong the life of all of his patients; this clearly included CPR. The two staff nurses echoed Dr. Beaudette's points and suggested they were certain that at least five or six nurses would leave RCNH rather than carry out a DNR policy.

Mr. Sturtevant then indicated that during the past week he had received many phone calls about this issue; to no one's surprise, the discussion had gone public. He had received a lengthy letter from the local "right to life" organization arguing strongly against RCNH adopting any form of a DNR policy, suggesting that it was "a scandal making people make this choice." They suggested they might even go so far as to organize demonstrations at the facility, should such a decision be made.

Along similar lines, Bill had heard more than once from a reporter for the only statewide daily newspaper, the *New Hampshire Register*, a paper considered to be controversial, highly conservative, and very influential. The reporter suggested that the only reason RCNH was considering implementing a DNR policy was to "clear out nonpaying patients so you can admit more private pay people." He planned an investigative report on the facility, its financing, and its operations. He also planned to attend all future meetings on the subject.

Shortly after having heard from the reporter, two key members of the Board of Commissioners called Bill to express their views. One commissioner commented that he had heard about all of this from the *Register* reporter (a contact which had upset him to begin with), and were the facility to implement a DNR policy, he would be forced to reconsider his long-standing commitment toward favorable appropriations. As he stated it, "This is a public place. What other choice do a lot of our residents have? If they can't count on the county home to take care of them for as long as possible, who can they count on? It's not like these folks have lots of resources; they can't pack up and go to another facility."

The second commissioner indicated that she was wholeheartedly in favor of a DNR policy for "both ethical and financial reasons, although the former are much more important on this issue."

Comments from around the room were divided, with a slight majority of the participants seeming to favor implementing a written DNR policy. The director of pastoral care at RCNH, a local Methodist minister, had given the matter considerable thought and was somewhat torn on the issue. In short, he suggested that, "On balance, I lean toward establishing a facilitywide DNR policy. Not only does this approach more appropriately recognize the sanctity of human life, it also will help residents, family, and staff know where they stand. It can create incredible uncertainty not having a policy down in writing on an issue this important. People need to know what they can expect when they enter Rockingham Home."

The final speaker was a lawyer. Since RCNH had no ongoing relationship with an attorney, Bill had asked the management team to identify one with an interest and expertise in this area who would be willing to volunteer to assist the committee. The attorney identified, Gwen Newhouse, had worked with RCNH on many issues in the past, including several involving clinical policies. She was a respected professional, enjoyed excellent ties with the Board of Commissioners and the state legislature, and was a member of the ethics committee at a nearby hospital. In Ms. Newhouse's opinion, "You just can't have such a DNR policy at Rockingham County Nursing Home. As one of the commissioners stated previously, 'Where are opposed people going to go?' As several nurses have suggested, 'Such a policy might precipitate problems recruiting high quality staff; we might even lose some of our valued medical staff.' Where would we be then? Isn't it our job to save lives? Haven't we all taken some sort of oath to do that? I hate to imagine what's going to happen when this policy gets out in terms of public relations; I hate to imagine the possible lawsuits that residents' families might file. Don't implement the policy—you're opening up a hornet's nest.

"There's lots of legislative activity going on now at the national and state levels about patient self-determination, living wills, durable power of attorney, and the like. It's not settled yet. If we just wait for a couple of years, the issue will be settled by the courts."

It was clear that resolution was not going to be easy. In his closing summary, Bill noted, "It's really too bad we don't have an institutional ethics committee; this would be a perfect issue for it to tackle. But we are where we are, and we need this group to resolve this question and to recommend the direction in which we ought to move. I still contend we should have a written DNR policy—one way or the other—either RCNH does or does not resuscitate residents who suffer an arrest. Maybe we should take a middle of the road stance, evaluating each situation on a case by case basis. After all, there is a strong moral argument for giving each individual a choice as to whether he or she wants to be resuscitated, and under what circumstances. But then a facility as large as ours, with only a limited number of ACLS-certified staff, could have major administrative difficulties with this approach, and it could be very costly. Not to mention, given our staffing patterns, how could we ensure that residents have access to a staff member skilled in CPR within a minute or so of arresting? How could we ever ensure that everyone was treated fairly and equally?"

After a minute of silent contemplation, Bill continued, "Again, whatever we do, we must do something. And, that 'something' has to be a decision that we can all stand behind in terms of its ethical foundation, resident care, marketing, finance, relations with the commissioners, and on and on. We may even have to revisit our organizational mission statement to make sure that we remain consistent with it.

"If I may, I'd like to suggest that you, Clare, as chair of this committee, continue to carry the ball and put together a draft institutional policy on DNR and why don't we plan to review it two weeks from now? We'll meet and discuss your ideas; you'd better give us your draft about a week before the meeting so we'll have time to react to it."

Back in your office several hours later, as is your practice, you summarize the key issues and questions on your yellow pad. After a very brief lunch you begin to address the items on your list. Although it's not possible to please everybody on this one, you know it is necessary to take a side. But first, all related questions must carefully be considered.

What should be RCNH's formal written institutional DNR policy? What are the potential ethical implications and moral conflicts having a formal DNR policy might precipitate? On what ethical grounds can we justify and defend it? How can we be sure the policy, whatever it is, will be fair? How can we avoid charges of discrimination?

What are the negative implications of this policy and how can we avoid them? What impact might it have for residents and families? How will the community respond to it? What might be its effect on RCNH's image and public relations?

Will adoption of a formal DNR policy require us to review and perhaps revise our mission statement, goals, or operations? How will it affect staff morale? Will it affect staff retention and recruitment? Will it increase our legal liability?

From an institutional perspective, how might it affect our occupancy rate, payer mix, or both? What reactions might we expect from the state legislature, governor, or the executive branch? Should we prepare for significant reactions by any prominent special interest groups (e.g., religious bodies, advocacy groups, professional associations)? How can we avoid, or minimize, any potential negative political fallout? Will our decision affect our relationships with other nursing facilities, particularly the other county homes in the state and others operating within our service area, or other area providers (e.g., physicians, hospitals)?

Thinking back specifically to the case of Mrs. Quimby, how would our proposed policy have affected her case, if at all? And, finally, what are our plans for periodic review of the policy?

Note

1. This act was passed as part of the Omnibus Reconciliation Act of 1990 which became effective on December 1, 1991.

The Jewish Homes for the Aging: Whose Rights Do We Serve?

Miriam Cotler

Introduction

THIS CASE describes the process by which an ethics committee develops a family notification policy. The need for this particular policy grew out of instances in which residents did not want private health-related information revealed to relatives, but relatives, in turn, demanded to be informed.

The Case of Sophie

Sophie, an 89-year-old woman, has lived in the nursing home for over four years. While physically frail, she has been generally healthy and very independent. She is busy with social activities and enjoys the library. Her two children are very active on the facility's advisory board and involved in her life. Sophie has been the strength in the family, and is a very proud and private woman.

As Sophie developed vague but frightening symptoms, she began to worry about cancer and the implications of what she believed to be a terminal illness. She knows her fears may be premature, and does not want to worry her children or deal with their reactions until she is sure. Sophie has completed an advance directive and does not want aggressive treatment. She told physicians, nurses, and other staff not "to discuss my medical case with my children. I am not ready, and when or if I am, I will do

---

The name of the organization and the issues presented in this case are real. Names of people have been changed.

it. My daughter gets hysterical and my son wants to take over. They mean well, but I need to be concerned with myself at this time, not with them."

The children asked for, and expected, regular updates on Sophie's health status. They wanted to know why she was tired lately and why she had visited the facility's clinic. They asked direct questions, and believed they were not being given complete information in return. Lately, they have become demanding, threatening to call board members and donors, complaining to the medical director and the administrator, and generally badgering the staff.

The Case of Betty

Betty has had a long history of chronic illness and recently has developed new symptoms. Her husband knows tests have been completed and asked the nurses to call him with the results, and not to tell Betty. Betty consistently and clearly has instructed staff not to tell her husband. She says he is worried and frightened and Betty wants him protected.

Should the facility accede to the demands of relatives or residents? Are the badgering children within their moral and legal rights? Is the frightened, agonized husband the facility's responsibility? How should staff respond? How should the ethics committee respond?

The Facility

The Jewish Homes for the Aging (JHA) is an 875-bed, multilevel of care facility on two campuses in the San Fernando Valley of Los Angeles. It is university-affiliated, research-oriented, and has a long history of innovation in social and medical services. Some of these services include adjacent houses and condominiums for independent living, an active out-patient day program, and a special care unit for residents with Alzheimer's disease. There are very busy ancillary clinical services, as well as active social, recreational, religious, library, and other programs. Unless they are unable to do so for medical reasons, residents are expected to attend meals in the large, attractive dining room.

On-site medical care is provided by three full-time physicians and a panel of attending physicians and allied professionals; acute services are provided through an affiliation with a nearby community hospital. Short stay, post-hospital care is available only for facility residents. The facilities provide lifelong, graded-level living for persons who entered when they were ambulatory and cognitively unimpaired. Residents usually are admitted to board and care. The average age at admission is 86 years; it is 91 among residents.

Each resident is asked to review, think about, and then complete a durable power of attorney for health care. Upon a resident or family member's request, assistance is available to help them understand the purpose and mechanics of the document. Residents name a surrogate, and sometimes request that their families not be notified about medical decisions or other private information. Competent residents may instruct staff to this effect at any time.

As the name implies, the home is religiously affiliated with the Jewish community, but it also recognizes and respects the diversity of religious orientations and affiliations existing among residents. There is a history of attention to residents' social and emotional needs, and residents have long had active councils and participation on the ethics committee. This committee, which has met regularly for more than eight years, has a broad membership. In addition to residents, it is comprised of staff and community physicians, nurses, social workers, administrators, admissions staff, ombudsmen, board members, community and university-affiliated rabbis, academics, contracted and volunteer attorneys, and community volunteers.

The Problem Presented to the Ethics Committee

When the need for a family notification policy was first brought to the attention of the ethics committee, it did not appear to be a particularly controversial or complex issue. The committee chair was approached by several members of the clinical and administrative staff. Some were unhappy with current practices, some were in disagreement with other staff or residents' families, some were concerned about compliance with regulations. Each saw a somewhat different problem, and their perspectives reflected the various interests at stake. They assigned a different level of priority to the values of respect for privacy, compassion for family, and staff rights to work without badgering from relatives.

The legal imperative comes from the Omnibus Reconciliation Act of 1987 (OBRA '87), which contains several clauses intended to assure nursing facility residents' rights based on moral principles of self-determination and privacy. The regulations include instructions for facilities to respect and protect residents' privacy, include rights to refuse to notify families and others about medical diagnosis, prognosis, and treatment options. But family members have, and often exercise, considerable power; they can and will put pressure on facilities to get this information.

Many medical, religious, nursing, and social service staff do not, or do not wish to, honor the principles of residents' rights. They may identify with the relatives or feel that some information is potentially harmful to residents. At other times they make decisions based on expediency, and thus, fail to comply with the spirit or the letter of OBRA.

The Problem within the Ethics Committee

At first glance, the issue seemed clear: Residents have the right to make their own decisions, even though relatives might object. The committee just needed to develop a mechanism for compliance. The policy should protect the rights of competent residents, include procedures to address the needs and rights of impaired residents, encourage communication between residents and families, and show compassion toward family members who are excluded from information.

However, there was deep disagreement among members of the ethics committee about the relative importance of families' and residents' rights. There was also disagreement about the extent to which OBRA really applies to resident transfers to and from the hospital and the implications of minor changes in residents' decision-making capacities. Committee members needed to understand the various political interests involved and the clinical issues related to competence. Ultimately, the province and role of the ethics committee itself were scrutinized.

The Problem as Perceived by Committee Members

The following categorization of committee members is presented as a means of summarizing viewpoints. It does not adequately reflect the complexity of the various positions. For example, some physicians identify strongly with families, and some board members are more sympathetic to residents than to families. The committee's problem is to resolve conflict and find compromise based on legal and moral principles. Members can be among the following:

1. *Residents' rights advocates.* The clinical staff on the committee (physicians, nurses, and social workers) generally agree that competent residents have a right to privacy with respect to his or her medical information. However, they feel harassed by families, especially when the resident is competent and wishes privacy. There is also conflict when the resident is not competent and has named a surrogate who is not a member of the family. Nursing staff may feel sorry for relatives, but these situations also interfere with their work.

2. *Families' rights advocates.* This group sees a trade-off between resident privacy and compassion for concerned families. These interests often are championed by the religious leaders involved, board members with parents in the home, and community

representatives. They recognize that the family members' interests are based on deep involvement and commitment, and they may believe the resident involved is acting unwisely.

3. *Compromisers.* These committee members tend to be administrators or members of the clinical management team who place priority on complying with regulations. They try to convince family members of the wisdom of the policy concerned. These persons may be seen as straddling the fence. They argue for a limited interpretation of the role of the ethics committee and try to address religious and board member interests.

Given these different approaches, the ethics committee has decided it needs to develop a policy endorsing the principles of resident self-determination within the framework of appropriate medical, social, and institutional care, as well as a family notification policy.

Marlton Nursing Home: To Tell or Not to Tell?

Bonnie S. Kantor and Gerald N. Cohn

Introduction

CAROL STERN, the director of nursing, sat quietly in David Allen's office, her supervisor, and listened as he finished what he had to say.

David Allen: "As executive director, I have to look beyond the resident we are discussing and evaluate any decisions made in the larger context of the policies of Marlton Nursing Home. We have to look at the medical facts, we have to consider the family and attending physician as well as the resident, we have to listen to the concerns of the nursing staff, and, we have to be sensitive to our community. Unfortunately, these perspectives do not add up to a clear decision. In reality, they contradict each other at several levels."

While Carol agreed, she felt that in her role as nursing supervisor she had to request a case review. The question important to her was who would conduct the review. The current options were a newly formed bioethics committee and a part-time medical director. If the rights of the resident, in this case Bernie Steinberg, were not respected, the nursing staff would feel that their professional ethics were being compromised. If the expressed wishes of the family and admitting physician were not respected, the nursing home could suffer in other ways.

This case is based on an incident that happened to a real resident in a real facility. However, the name of the individual, the organization, and some events have been changed to assure anonymity.

Carol could not afford to take this decision lightly, both as a manager and from a medical ethics point of view. She expressed her concerns to David Allen, and asked what he planned to do.

The Case of Bernie Steinberg

Sally Kish, admissions coordinator, personally assisted Bernie Steinberg, age 72, through the admissions process at Marlton Nursing Home. Bernie had arrived in a private ambulance from nearby Lakeland Hospital; his daughter, Susan Mills, had family responsibilities and could not be there. Susan gave the nursing home instructions over the telephone to proceed without her. She would be by later that evening.

As part of the admission process at Marlton, new residents are administered a series of diagnostic tests to assess their cognitive abilities. Bernie's test scores indicated that he was alert, oriented, and functional. Had his diagnosis showed him to be disoriented or incompetent, the admissions process would have stopped until a family member or guardian could be called to complete advance directives.

Sally reviewed the advance directives and consent for resuscitation policy forms with Bernie, to which he expressed surprise.

Bernie Steinberg: "I don't understand. Why would you ask me such a question? I'm Jewish."

Sally Kish: "Mr. Steinberg, it's not always a simple issue. Resuscitation can be traumatic for patients and families, and the long-term outcome is never known for sure. You don't have to decide this now. Perhaps we can wait until your family is here. That would be best."

Bernie Steinberg: "That's not necessary. Jewish law is very clear on the subject of resuscitation. Living is not our choice, it is our responsibility."

At that point, Bernie signed the advance directives (see Exhibit 9.1), indicating that all forms of intervention should be used and that he should be resuscitated in the event of cardiac arrest.

History and Subsequent Actions

Bernie Steinberg survived German concentration camps in the 1940s and after several years in resettlement camps came to the United States, settling in Marlton, Colorado. He married, had a successful business as a kosher butcher, and was active in his synagogue. When his wife died ten years ago, he grieved deeply, but refused to move in with his only child, Susan, and her family. Bernie and Susan maintained their very close relationship, and he maintained his independence.

Several years ago, Bernie began to exhibit symptoms of pallor, cachexia, ascites, black tarry stools, anemia, and abdominal aching, pressure,

Exhibit 9.1   Consent for Resuscitation Policy

The Marlton Nursing Home defines a DNR (Do Not Resuscitate) order as a medical decision not to begin CPR (Cardiac-pulmonary resuscitation) on a Resident if the Resident has experienced the sudden cessation of breathing and heartbeat due to a possible heart attack or stroke.

A Resident who stops breathing and whose vital signs cease to appear as a consequence of the natural dying process, would not be administered CPR. In these circumstances, the emergency squad would not be called and the Resident would not be transported to the hospital.

The option of a DNR order will be discussed with a capable Resident and family prior to or upon admission by a member of the Social Work Staff. A Resident and family will be asked to complete a DNR decision form which will be part of the Resident's permanent medical record.

In the case of a Resident who is incompetent to make an informed decision concerning DNR: if the physician wishes to order DNR status on an incompetent Resident who is terminally ill or in an irreversible coma, the physician can do so by discussing DNR with the Resident's family or responsible party, and documenting the discussion and the decision in the physician progress notes. The DNR order will be written as a physician order on the Resident's chart.

The Resident and family have the right to change DNR order or initiate a DNR order at any time. The change must be made in writing by the use of the DNR decision form.

A DNR order will be documented in the Resident's chart by the Resident's physician.

Resident Name _____

_____ I/we request a DNR (Do Not Resuscitate) order to be written by my physician in my medical chart.

_____ I/we request that all life-saving procedures, IE-CPR, be initiated if I stop breathing.

_____ I/we am/are unable to decide at this time pending further discussion with the physician. I/we understand that all life-saving procedures will be initiated if I stop breathing.

_____   _____
Family Member/Responsible Party   Resident

_____   _____
Date   Witness

and dull cramps. His diagnosis was colorectal cancer. As the cancer progressed, Bernie developed weakness, fatigue, exertional dippnea, vertigo, and eventually diarrhea, weight loss, anorexia, and occasional vomiting. He was aggressively treated for the cancer, and had been in and out of remission since his initial diagnosis. Recently, Bernie had had surgery to resection the sigmoid colon and the mesentery, as well as repeated radiation treatments.

Following surgery Bernie was disoriented and needed constant care and medication administration, as well as subacute short-term rehabilitation. This level of post-surgery care was not covered in a hospital. The family's personal physician, Dr. Joseph Dish, Susan, and Bernie had agreed that he should continue his recuperation at the Marlton Nursing Home, and expected him to return home in about six weeks. Susan was a board member at Marlton and had been actively involved in the building fund for the new, modern facility. Prior to leaving the hospital, additional diagnostic tests were performed, although the results were not yet available.

Soon after Bernie entered Marlton Nursing Home, his health deteriorated and he showed early symptoms of dysphagia and weight loss. The dysphagia became constant, with pain on swallowing, coughing, and glossopharyngeal neuralgia. Dr. Dish did not act on these new symptoms, but continued waiting for the results of tests run. In the meantime, Bernie kept asking the nursing staff what was wrong. They told him they were waiting to find out. When the results came back, they confirmed Dr. Dish's suspicions: Bernie Steinberg was suffering from esophageal cancer. Dr. Dish arranged to meet with Susan.

Dr. Dish: "Susan, since we're longtime friends, I'm going to be completely honest with you. No treatment will completely eradicate this form of cancer. Surgical treatment can be radical and involves resection of the esophagus, reconstruction to maintain a passageway for food, colon bypass grafts, prosthetic tubes, and subsequent chemotherapy. Complications are common, particularly at Bernie's age. My recommendation is that your father be made comfortable and given adequate nutrition. I do not recommend surgery or other invasive measures."

Susan was extremely upset. After a few minutes, she was able to respond:

Susan: "I agree with you, I don't want my father to suffer any longer. As he fought to stay alive in Europe, he'd probably fight now, but I don't want that. I want my father to be comfortable, that's all."

They discussed this further and agreed that Bernie should not be told of his advanced diagnosis. They both believed that if he knew, he

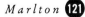

would most assuredly try to fight the disease at all costs to himself and his family.

Dr. Dish: "I'll inform the nursing and medical staff that they are not to tell Bernie about his condition. You'll have to complete new advance directives, including a 'Do Not Resuscitate' (DNR) order. These will override the previous orders your father signed."

The next day, Susan filled out new advance directives, noting the family's decisions and the attending physician's concurrence for a DNR order. Susan gave these to the head nurse on the floor and said they superseded any previous orders on file. The new directives indicated that, when the time came, Bernie was only to be given oxygen, intravenous hydration, and analgesics to keep him comfortable.

The new directives generated a great deal of anger and confusion among the nursing staff. They all had gotten to know Bernie, and affectionately referred to him as a "fighter" because of his indomitable belief that he could "lick anything." They felt that no decision could be made without Bernie's participation, and that these new directives were in conflict with his resident rights. Perhaps most importantly, the directives forbid them to respond directly to any questions Bernie asked about his condition. They felt that all of this compromised their professional code of ethics.

Because her nursing staff was upset, the head floor nurse consulted Carol Stern, the director of nursing, for further clarification. The nurses felt these orders hindered their ability to provide quality care. They also strongly felt that they could not withhold nutrition. One of the student nurses knew that this type of cancer had been treated with some success using a feeding tube during radiation therapy. The floor staff discussed this with the medical director, Dr. Jones, who agreed that something might be done. He felt that while the cancer would not be cured, intervention would make the resident more comfortable as the cancer progressed. Dr. Jones was concerned with the decisions of the admitting physician and the family. In addition, they all felt that the policies and procedures of the nursing home needed clarification.

Carol called Susan and asked if they could meet that afternoon. Susan rearranged her day for an early afternoon meeting.

Carol Stern: "I'm sorry about your father's condition. I just heard the diagnosis was esophagal cancer. My nurses tell me you and Dr. Dish discussed treatment, and that you completed advance directives for your father. Were you aware your father completed these forms just two weeks ago when he entered the nursing home? He asked that all means be taken to seek treatment."

Susan Mills: "I know my father completed advance directives during admission, but his medical condition has changed. You aren't suggesting that the old directives are valid, are you? I'm his daughter and I want the best for him. Based on the change in his diagnosis, Dr. Dish and I concur that treatment should be discontinued. This is our decision. Dr. Dish feels nothing can be done to cure my father. Knowing this, I will not permit any interventions, except to make sure he is comfortable. I've written this all in the advance directives and Dr. Dish noted it in my father's chart."

Carol Stern: "I've gone over Marlton's policy regarding advance directives. They are currently being revised, but they still stand. They state that as long as your father is competent, only he can change his advance directives. He really must be consulted. Also, his treating physician should review any major changes in his diagnosis with the medical director.

"We just want what is best for you and your father. Try to understand how difficult this makes it for the nurses caring for your father. Perhaps if you talk with your father, he may agree with you."

Susan became extremely angry and suggested that Carol Stern may have just overstepped her bounds. Carol hastened to assure her she was only acting on behalf of the nursing staff and following policy in bringing these issues to the family.

Susan Stern: "My father is in constant pain, and yet he would never listen to me, nor would he accept his condition. To me, that isn't competent. That's it. Please see that my orders are respected. My father is to be told nothing of his medical condition. Is that clear? I do not expect my orders to be ignored. Hereafter, you may direct any questions or concerns to our physician, Dr. Dish."

Carol: "I'm sorry. However, as I understand, your father cannot be excluded from this decision as long as he is competent. His original advance directives cannot be ignored."

Susan left the room, clearly agitated. Less than an hour later, David Allen called Carol into his office.

David Allen: "Carol, Susan Mills just called me about her father. She's extremely angry and feels you and the staff are pressuring her. I think in this case, you should have come to me first and let me talk with Susan. When we admit a resident to the facility we also admit the family, and I feel we should balance the needs of both. Beside being Bernie's only living relative, she is one of the major supporters of Marlton, a board member, and helped build this facility. How she feels is important to all of us. And how she feels right now is that we are not respecting her and her physician's decisions, which were difficult enough to make.

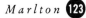

"Susan freely admits to me that if told of his new bout with cancer, her father would try to fight it like he has everything in his life. Because of this and his deterioration in symptoms, she feels he is not competent to make any further decisions."

Carol Stern: "I'm sympathetic to the family, but I cannot agree. I'm not just speaking as an individual, but as a staff representative. Everything we are being asked to do contradicts our commitment to quality care, resident rights, and medical ethics. Can't Dr. Jones, as medical director, consult with Dr. Dish for clarification?

"What you may not realize is, although Bernie's physical and emotional health have deteriorated since his admission, he is still alert and takes an interest in everything going on, especially regarding his health. I feel that our own policy demands we inform him. In fact, we have to consult him in order to change his resuscitation orders.

"Current regulations state that 'Except in a medical emergency or when a resident is incompetent, a facility must consult with the resident immediately when there is a significant change in the resident's physical, mental, or psychosocial status.' Are we debating issues of emotional and mental competency, or whether different forms of cancer are considered a change in medical status?"

David Allen was not surprised that a situation such as this had arisen. In his mind, the nursing home was "prime" for this kind of incident. He understood Carol Stern's concern about resident rights and medical policy concerning advance directives. But to him, the issues were even more serious. Over the last several years, he had seen Marlton go from 20 percent admissions for subcute care patients needing to complete recuperation following hospitalization or chronic illness, to over 60 percent. With this had come the need to provide stronger medical direction and more choices about medical interventions.

The current medical director at Marlton, Dr. Jones, served in that capacity without direct payment from the facility. His only compensation came from his patients' reimbursements. Admitting physicians maintain responsibility for their own patients, with few guidelines imposed by Marlton.

David Allen: "In terms of medical review, Dr. Kevin Jones does not have the authority to override the attending physician's orders. Perhaps policy in this area could be developed for future cases. However, at this time, Dr. Dish has the authority for this case.

"In terms of Bernie's rights, I will meet with Dr. Dish and Susan to discuss this further. I don't think you should call a meeting of the Bioethics Committee. The committee has only existed for six months, has met only once, and has not undergone the proposed education programs which would prepare it for case review responsibilities. Also, Susan and Dr. Dish are members of the committee and would feel it was a breech of confidentiality to discuss this case.

"Please work with your nursing staff and let them know that the case is being reviewed internally. Until my review is completed, they are to abide by the family's decision."

Facility Description

Marlton Nursing Home was established in 1954 as a private, nonprofit, religiously affiliated, long-term care facility for persons needing full-time nursing care. With strong, continuous community support and the generosity of many individuals, a new state-of-the-art facility was recently constructed, with increased capacity for 180 residents.

The nursing home has a 60 percent Medicaid occupancy rate. A large development campaign annually helps to underwrite the cost of care. Costs are high at Marlton because of the excellent care provided, the new facility, the availability of private rooms for each resident, and high staff-to-resident ratios far exceeding minimum standards. Everyone was proud that staff turnover was significantly lower than the 50 percent rate reported nationwide.

Facility Medical Policies and Procedures

David Allen, executive director, was aware that a more comprehensive admissions procedure to the nursing home was needed, one that could include family and patient conferences to review facility policies, advance directives, and other areas of concern. The advance directives and resuscitation forms currently used were poorly written and extremely vague, particularly in identifying the wide range of medical technologies available today and determining whether or not they would be used (see Exhibit 9.1).

These directives, however, were only part of the problem, which included the need for new medical policies and procedures and strong physician leadership. The board of directors had previously tabled discussion of these issues in place of other, more pressing issues, particularly increasing community financial support. The community was proud of the new facility and the board wanted to build on this support while enthusiasm was high.

The director of Nursing, Carol Stern, took it upon herself to share her views about medical policies and procedures with the board and David Allen. The forms used during admission were of particular concern, since the admissions department reported to her. In a recent memo,

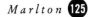

she noted the need to revise the advance directives in line with research and available models in the field. The materials they were currently using made no distinctions between the resident and family, had no place for the input or verification of the physician, and did not attempt to define such critical issues as "competent" and "life-threatening." Scheduled reviews of advance directives were not part of regular operations.

The only structure for personnel mediation was directly with the executive director. Carol felt this was a potential area of conflict; mediation should be a joint process with the medical director, a bioethics committee, and the executive director.

Development of the Bioethics Committee

When Carol Stern came to Marlton Nursing Home two years ago a "Medical Committee" was in place that was charged with reviewing medical policies. While the bylaws for the committee recommended bimonthly meetings, the committee met irregularly—twice in the last calendar year, with fewer than five members out of 15 attending.

During the process of establishing her new program goals, Carol reviewed related policies and procedures. Her primary goal was to respect the rights of patients and assure that all patients received a high quality of care. The review process revealed just how little medical supervision and direction the nursing staff received, and the lack of strong medical procedures for case review and medical policies.

Carol asked David Allen to petition the Board of Directors to disband the Medical Committee and, in its place, establish a Bioethics Committee. She felt this was needed because the expansion of medical technology into nursing homes posed difficult ethical questions, many of which had to be consistent with the diverse cultural and religious backgrounds of the residents. The Medical Committee, aside from being nearly defunct, did not address the more comprehensive issues facing this facility. To support her request, she prepared a "research memo" for her supervisor, found in Exhibit 9.2.

David Allen was delighted with the thoroughness of Carol's memo and strongly supported her request at the next board meeting. The board was just as enthusiastic in its support, and unanimously voted to disband the Medical Committee and establish, in its place, a Bioethics Committee. The board saw the Bioethics Committee not only as important to maintaining the high quality of care at the nursing home, but also as a public relations vehicle for letting the community witness the high level of responsibility that the nursing home takes toward its residents and their families. The board felt the Bioethics Committee could also enhance its fundraising efforts.

Exhibit 9.2 Research Memo

TO: David Allen, Executive Director
FROM: Carol Stern, Director of Nursing
SUBJECT: Medical Directorship and Bioethics Committee

As I've personally witnessed in various other short- and long-term care facilities in the country, bioethics committees are increasingly being utilized to supplement strong medical direction. The usefulness of these committees have paralleled the growing number of residents who are older and sicker than ever before.

Marlton Nursing Home would benefit from expanding the role of medical director and by developing a bioethics committee. The medical director should establish medical policies, with emphasis on the care of subacute residents. Such policy, communicated to attending and consultant physicians, would help us achieve the highest quality of care possible. The medical director would also provide direction to the bioethics committee, which would develop ethical guidelines and conduct case reviews.

The bioethics committee would bring together a diversity of personal and professional perspectives to add to the analysis of problems. I suggest it be given three primary responsibilities. It should (1) develop strong staff and community education programs around bioethical issues; (2) serve as an advisory group to conduct and mediate reviews of problematic cases; and (3) support and contribute to policy development for Marlton.

Educational programs could help sensitize staff and families about important ethical issues, potential conflicts, and methods of resolution. Case reviews would be conducted on a random selection basis to supplement educational programs, and on an as needed basis when requested by the medical director or nursing staff.

Policy formation would perhaps be the most important task for the committee, as it would have the most direct effect on the staff, on residents, and on their families. Initial efforts should address a complete revision of the current advance directives, resuscitation orders, definitions of "competency," and other areas in which institutional policies have ethical implications. In this way, when case reviews do come about, the Bioethics Committee will have established guidelines to define the limits of ethically acceptable and legally permissible behaviors.

Please let me know of your decision so that I can continue planning program goals for nursing and admissions.

The charge of the committee was fourfold: education, case review, consent for research, and policymaking. Composition of the 20-person committee was broad based to assure its success, and to highlight its importance to the nursing home and the community at large. David Allen and Carol Stern would serve on the committee, which would be headed by Kevin Jones, the medical director. Additional members would include attorneys, educators, physicians from a variety of specialties, and others from the community, including a consultant from a nearby university.

The first meeting of the Bioethics Committee was highly successful, with over 75 percent of the members attending. At that meeting, the committee voted to table development of a full-time medical director position until the next fiscal year. The second meeting was scheduled for the following month, at which time Bernie Steinberg's case would be reviewed. Carol wondered, however, how his case would be handled in the meantime.

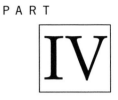
Operations Challenges

10

Good Shepherd Village:
Interdisciplinary Team Development

William E. Aaronson and Jacqueline S. Zinn

Introduction

JOHN EVANS had just left a meeting of the Geriatric Assessment and Care Planning Team of the Good Shepherd Village (GSV). The discussions at the team meeting had surprised and bewildered him. John felt he was the object of downright hostility. This was only John's sixth month in the position of director of health services for GSV, but already he was becoming a center of controversy for his "radical" views. John recently had returned to his native rural Pennsylvania community to assume this position. Although he had been gone for more than ten years, John knew the community remained staunchly conservative and wary of new ideas. In contrast to the local residents, John expected the professionals at GSV to be more cosmopolitan and accepting of his ideas. Integrated delivery systems had become the ideal among health service providers in the city he had just left, and nothing better exemplified an integrated delivery system than a continuing care retirement community (CCRC). However, the health professionals at GSV resisted implementation of the proposed changes in team procedures. Most adamantly opposed to the changes was Dr. Aaron Schmidt, the medical director.

John began having serious doubts about his decision to return home. He had left a well-paid position as associate executive director of a

This case is based on two vignettes that appeared in Aaronson, W. and R. Neuhaus, "The Professional Team: Core Technology for Long-Term Care," curriculum module in *Learning the Continuum: AUPHA Modules for Management Education*, pp. 50–57, Office of Long-term Care and Aging, AUPHA, Arlington, Virginia, 1989, and the consulting and research experience of the authors.

university-affiliated teaching nursing home. Despite the progressive atmosphere at the teaching nursing home, the opportunity at GSV had appeared attractive, and besides, he felt a sense of obligation to care for his ailing parents. His instincts told him GSV was already an outstanding retirement community and with the progressive ideas he brought, GSV could become the best of many outstanding CCRCs in the state.

Background

The Good Shepherd Village is a multilevel continuing care retirement community located on 300 acres in a semirural community within easy driving distance of Philadelphia. Good Shepherd is affiliated with the Lutheran Synod and Lutheran Social Services. The current campus configuration was completed in 1987. Reverend Kathleen Mueller was appointed chair of the board that year. Bill Wagner, a highly respected retirement community executive, assumed the executive director position in 1979.

Continuing Care at GSV

The retirement community contains 550 independent living units, including one- and two-bedroom apartments and single story, detached cottages, 120 licensed nursing care beds, 30 licensed personal care beds and 20 congregate living studio units. Besides the physical facilities, GSV maintains comprehensive health, social, rehabilitative, and recreational services, and operates a Medicare-certified home health agency. The agency provides services to residents of surrounding communities, and also to the residents of GSV. Thus, GSV offers a self-contained continuum of care to residents entering the community.

Residents pay a substantial entrance fee (see Table 10.1) when entering independent or congregate living. They may make occasional use of personal or nursing facility care at no additional charge. Medicare, supplemented by Medigap policies, frequently covers short stays in full. However, if residents enter the nursing facility on a long-stay basis, they pay the nursing facility discounted rate (see Table 10.2). The discounted rate is considerably below the cost of private nursing home care, but is greater than the rate for a full-service plan contract in independent living.

Prospective residents are offered a variety of cost and accommodation options. The entrance fees are as low as $55,000 for the congregate care studio apartments to as high as $155,000 for a cottage with a carport. GSV can easily resell the cottages and the deluxe two-bedroom apartments to persons on a waiting list. However, congreate care studio

Table 10.1 Entrance and Service Plan Charges

| Accommodation | Entrance Fee | Monthly Fee* | | |
		Full Service	Modified	Independent
Cottage with carport 50 units	$155,000	$1,550	$1,000	$500
Two-bedroom deluxe 120 units	$125,000	$1,450	$950	$400
Two-bedroom standard 80 units	$112,500	$1,400	$900	$350
One-bedroom deluxe 200 units	$94,500	$1,350	$850	$400
One-bedroom standard 100 units	$84,500	$1,200	$800	$350
Studio apartment congregate	$55,000	$1,450	n/a	n/a

* Rates based on single occupancy. Spouses add $950 to full service and $475 to modified service plan.

Table 10.2 Nursing Facility Charges*

	Semi-Private Full Charge	Semi-Private Discount**	Private Full Charge	Private Discount**
Personal care	n/a	n/a	$2,571	$1,928
Nursing facility	$3,176	$2,382	$3,479	$2,609

* Rates are published on a per diem basis. Monthly rates are estimated based on 30.25 days per month.
** The continuing care discount is the rate set in accordance with the continuing care contract entered into by the resident at the time of admission to Good Shepherd Village. Persons entering the nursing center from outside of GSV pay full charges.

apartments are not as marketable. Minimal supervision is provided in these studio apartments, which are attached to the personal care unit.

Residents entering the independent living units also have a choice of three service packages. The full-service contract includes ten meals per week in the Village Inn, in-home personal services, attendant services for activity of daily living (ADL) assistance, and an upgraded recreation package including a choice of season tickets to the Philadelphia Orchestra or attendance at off-Broadway performances in Philadelphia. The modified plan includes fewer meals and amenities. Attendant services are provided at a discounted rate. The independent plan includes no meals, but includes access to planned recreation. Access to attendant services at full charge is guaranteed. However, the price paid by GSV residents is lower than the cost of comparable services in the community. Personal care and nursing service access at the discounted rates is guaranteed to all, whatever plan is selected.

The availability of attendant services is a particularly marketable aspect of the continuing care contract. Attendant services indicate GSV's commitment to maintain residents' independence as long as possible. However, the attendant service clause increases financial risk to GSV because they are expensive, and the need for them has been increasing as residents age in place. Thus, there is a strong incentive to classify residents as long-stay nursing home patients whenever possible. Once a person's need for attendant services crosses a certain threshold, they might be better served in personal care or in the nursing facility.

Residents admitted to personal care pay no entrance fee, but do pay the full per diem charge in the nursing care facility, and are not guaranteed access. Residents may also enter the nursing care facility directly, based on availability.

The nursing facility is Medicaid-certified. Continued certification following the development of the retirement community was necessary due to the holdovers from the old home who continued to be covered by Medicaid. With spenddown by persons admitted directly into the nursing facility possible, continued Medicaid certification was essential. Medicaid certification also provides a safety net for GSV residents who outlive their assets. No one has ever been dismissed from GSV for lack of funds. Management monitors the proportion of Medicaid patient days closely and keeps them at a level compatible with the financial objectives of GSV. GSV also has accumulated a substantial indigent care endowment, the income from which subsidizes care of persons residing in personal care.

The New Health Services Director

The position of director of health services was created as a result of the increasing medical need of residents of GSV. Average age on admission increased from 71 in 1982 to the current average of 77 years. Longevity of residents seemed to increase every year as well, with four residents in the nursing facility now who are older than 100, and a high proportion of residents older than 85 years and frail. The need for greater coordination of health services was evident. Service duplication and overlap was costly, and adversely affected quality.

John came to the position of director of health services at Good Shepherd with exceptional credentials, including a joint Master of Health Administration and Master of Science in Nursing (MHA/MSN) degree from an accredited eastern college.

The director of health services was to be responsible for the provision of all health services in this multilevel campus. GSV provided what had been felt to be a fairly comprehensive health care package designed to keep people healthy and maintain their functional independence. Everything from a fitness center to coordinated physician care was available to the residents of the independent living units. The health, rehabilitation, and social service staffs conducted parallel assessments of residents in independent living. Concerns about resident health or safety triggered a full assessment. Residents unable to care for their personal needs might require more services or a higher level of residential care. Following assessments, the multidisciplinary health care team would meet, discuss the assessments and make a recommendation to the medical director.

John knew that the new position would be challenging, but he never expected it to be quite this challenging. As an associate executive director at a teaching nursing home, John had supervised clinical services and managed the teaching affiliation agreements with the university's academic departments of nursing, physical therapy, and therapeutic recreation. Two students from each discipline were assigned to each floor on a seven-week rotation. They learned to work in teams, and their nursing home preceptors took great pride in their ability to model a team spirit. Based on his experience, John had not been exposed to differences and conflicts among health and health-related professions, and was ill-prepared to deal with the level of discomfort that existed among the GSV staff. Their cordiality toward each other, while genuine on an interpersonal level, covered a more basic mistrust and misunderstanding of each other's professional responsibilities.

Level of Care Decisions and Team Effectiveness

Prior to the creation of the position of director of health services, Dr. Schmidt was nominally in charge of the multidisciplinary team and supervised the rehabilitation departments. The social service and recreation departments reported to the executive director. Based on the recommendation of the multidisciplinary team, the medical director and the executive director made the level of care decisions. In theory, such decisions were based on medical need, however, nursing home certification is less clear in a continuing care retirement community, such as GSV, than for persons living at home. The availability of attendant services meant that residents with ADL deficits could remain in their units when they required help. The support network of neighbors and professional staff was also a source of strength for residents as their personal independence began to slip away.

Unfortunately, there was a strong incentive to move residents to higher levels of care when the cost of providing care in their units increased. The full-service contract provided for unlimited use of services. The modified contract provided for a number of in-home services and deep discounts on those not directly covered by the contract. Very few residents opt for the pay-as-you-go option, which provides no services and more limited discounts on in-home services. The "free" care and the deep discounts had become problematic because the home health service was experiencing increasing community demand. Since these nonskilled care and personal care services were provided at full charge to surrounding communities, services provided under the contract carried an opportunity cost of lost profits. The inability of GSV to recruit enough staff to serve both programs made this a problem. Chronic shortages of skilled professionals and certified nursing assistants made it difficult to stay fully staffed.

Financially, besides the increased revenues available when residents stayed in the nursing facility, there was a substantial waiting list for all independent living unit types, except for the smallest one-bedroom units. Each of the independent living units, thus, could be "resold" when it was released from use by a current resident. In theory, long-stay nursing facility residents could return to independent living; in reality, no long-stay resident had ever returned to independent living. However, several long-stay residents had transferred to personal care. Thus, there were strong incentives to transfer residents permanently to the nursing facility once they required more extensive in-home supportive services.

Despite John's short tenure at GSV, he was certain that he had accurately diagnosed the organizational problems he faced in managing the health services of the residents. The issues were twofold: (1) the economics of the continuing care contract influenced level of care decisions more than was necessary; and (2) the multidisciplinary team was not functioning as a team, resulting in fragmented service delivery and ineffective care management.

John was deeply concerned about the potential effects on team decisions posed by economic incentives. While the team was unlikely to be swayed directly by economic incentives, the disarray and lack of leadership under Dr. Schmidt and Mr. Wagner led to the team's acquiescence in most levels of care decisions. According to Louise Richards, the chief physical therapist, there had never been an egregious example of a transfer for which there was no justification. John also believed that the ineffectiveness of the team was adversely affecting quality of care and increasing financial risk to GSV. Improved team function should enhance prevention efforts and reduce future morbidities. With fewer morbidities, residents would face less risk of a high-cost nursing facility stay.

Under the current approach, the Medical, Rehabilitation (physical therapist, occupational therapist, and speech pathologist), Social Services, and Nursing staffs each submitted separate evaluations on the potential for a resident to continue to live independently. Based on these evaluations, each of the team participants developed a care and rehabilitation plan. The therapists carried out treatment modalities once the attending physician for that resident approved and ordered any necessary treatments. The team would then meet and recommend a permanent placement to the medical director and the executive director.

Based on his previous experience and his personal philosophy of care, John preferred a more dynamic group process in which team members would identify resident health problems jointly and develop a set of objectives for each problem. He felt that focusing on client function and developing care plans designed to maintain optimal function would circumvent the level of care issue and prevent premature transfer to the nursing center. John had worked hard to gain support for his team development plan. However, more accurate geriatric assessments and more effective care plans could result in fewer admissions to the nursing facility and higher costs in the independent living units as more health-related services were provided.

John received the most support for his proposal to develop a more coordinated and integrated interdisciplinary team with expanded care management responsibilities from the board chair, Reverend Kathleen Mueller. She strongly supported the idea because it appeared more likely to result in a holistic approach to care. She also felt it gave visiting clergy a more cogent role in care planning, something she felt to be important in a religiously affiliated community.

There was considerable dissent among the board members over this issue. The loudest dissent, however, came from the executive director, Bill Wagner, who felt this approach inhibited the quick action required when someone's health deteriorated rapidly. The board ultimately agreed with Reverend Mueller and pressed Mr. Wagner to carry out the Geriatric Assessment and Care Planning Team approach. John was given the responsibility of organizing the team.

New Supervisory Responsibilities

The purpose of the new position was to relieve Dr. Schmidt of supervisory responsibility within the functionally organized rehabilitation

Figure 10.1 Good Shepherd Village Organization Chart

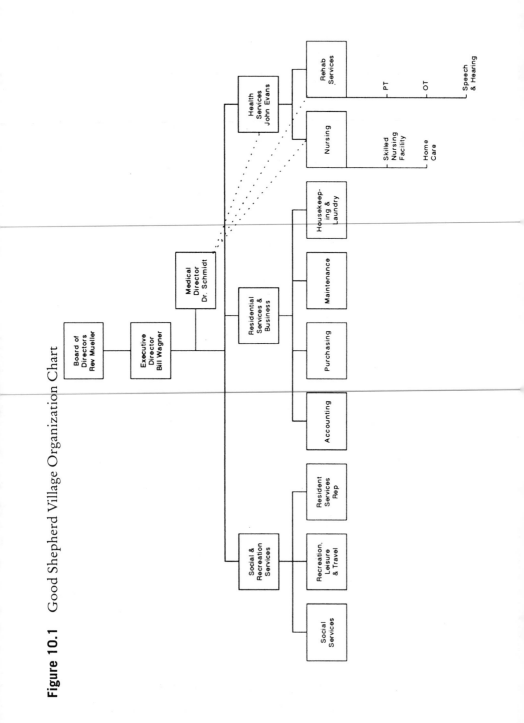

departments. It was also intended to provide greater administrative oversight over the nursing facility and home care departments. Figure 10.1 shows the new table of organization. The position of social and recreation services director was created, but not filled. Social and recreational services staff nominally reported to Bill Wagner, however, John became their supervisor de facto. Thus, John had supervisory authority over much of the professional staff at GSV.

John spoke to each of his immediate subordinates about the need to improve team functioning, and most of the meetings they held were similar in nature. John talked extensively about the merits of interdisciplinary cooperation and integration. He told each member of the staff that he hoped to work with them at improving functional assessments. The responses were almost all the same . . . polite silence, then each subordinate talked freely about his or her duties. All agreed that GSV was a great place to work. The residents were terrific and Dr. Schmidt was reasonable, for a physician. Bill Wagner did not interfere with their work. Maggie Newman, director of nursing, complained about communication between nursing staff and personal physicians. She added that Dr. Schmidt was helpful in getting the personal physicians to communicate with GSV professional staff. Maggie's biggest concern was over scheduling of rehabilitation appointments. Appointments were not coordinated between independent living and the nursing facility. Consequently, independent living residents occasionally were scheduled for therapies at the same time as nursing facility residents. This upset the independent living residents, who did not want to be reminded of the natural courses of their chronic illnesses.

The resident council echoed Maggie's concerns to John. The Resident Council chair told John that the staff at GSV couldn't be nicer. Recreational, nursing, and therapy staff were helpful and seemed competent. However, having just recovered from a fractured leg, he said it had appeared that each of the therapists didn't know what the others were doing. His fracture was compound, requiring surgery and extensive rehabilitation, and he seemed annoyed that he had to tell each therapist the same things he had told his doctor and the orthopedic surgeon. He wanted to know if anybody communicated. John realized that the Resident Council chair didn't know the difference between a physical and occupational therapist, that he thought they were all the same, as well as the "therapy" they were doing.

Louise Richards, chief physical therapist, was annoyed when John told her this anecdote. She said that residents frequently need instruction on the type of therapy they are receiving. She said, further, that physicians don't prepare residents adequately for therapy, and someone else has to explain the reasons for and expected results from therapy the doctor has ordered.

During his initial six months, John attended many multidisciplinary team meetings. Each was similar in structure, with each team member giving an evaluation summary and outlining changes in courses of treatment for their department. Team members were occasionally questioned about their assumptions or given some information they may not have been aware of. However, team meetings were not considered a place to debate the most important issues. Within six months John had formulated new team policies and procedures. He had developed a common assessment form and a new team meeting format, which he had put in writing and was preparing to circulate. He intended to provide in-service training to all staff who would be participating on the new interdisciplinary team. The team would now have a title, the Geriatric Assessment and Care Planning Team, and expanded responsibilities for the integration of resident care services. John was enthusiastic about his plan, and believed the professional staff would share his enthusiasm once they became fully aware of the changes he was introducing.

Bill Wagner remained skeptical of these changes, and approved the new procedures reluctantly. John held a meeting of all professional services staff, including Dr. Schmidt, wherein John handed each a packet of information and explained the new procedures and expectations. Dr. Schmidt objected that he would be unable to participate in many team meetings unless they could be more favorably scheduled. John wanted to implement the new procedures within three months, and asked the team to provide feedback as soon as possible so he could finalize the procedures. The deadline for submission to the board for approval was approaching. He reminded the staff that he had been directed to do this by Reverend Mueller, and that he expected only minor changes in the present document.

The Case of Mrs. Imelda White

The next meeting of the multidisciplinary team was the first opportunity to test the value of this new approach. However, the meeting became heated during a level of care decision for Mrs. Imelda White, a longtime resident. Mrs. White had been widowed four years ago and recently suffered a cerebrovascular accident (CVA) while attending the Palm Sunday service conducted by the Reverend Mueller. Reverend Mueller took an active interest in Mrs White's care following the incident, which added urgency to the team's responsibilities, and an unusual level of tension. The board chair's interest heightened the controversy over the impending level of care decision. Mrs. White currently was in a highly reputable rehabilitation hospital where she was undergoing intensive rehabilitation to restore as much function as possible.

Because of the stroke, Mrs. White had experienced a partial right hemiplegia, a slight swallowing dysphagia with an accompanying speech impediment, and slight memory loss. Her cognitive function was good, but her physical function left some question about her ability to remain mobile and independent. John was confident that Mrs. White, with continued rehabilitation, could probably return to independent living, however, Bill Wagner and Dr. Schmidt expressed serious reservations. They were also concerned about the staff's ability to provide the necessary level of in-home support, given her age, frailty, and disability. John felt that Bill Wagner may have had an ulterior motive in suggesting that Mrs. White give up her popular two-bedroom deluxe apartment.

John had visited Mrs. White in the rehabilitation hospital, where he had an extensive discussion with members of the hospital's rehabilitation team. They believed that Mrs. White would have been unable to live at home alone, but should do well in the supportive environment of GSV. Mrs. White said that her goal was to return to her apartment as soon as possible. Given the level of cooperation expressed by the hospital rehabilitation team and Mrs. White's desire to return to independent living, John believed the Geriatric Assessment and Care Planning team should be willing to participate in a comprehensive functional assessment. The assessment was to begin while she was in the hospital, and to continue when she returned to the nursing unit for ongoing rehabilitation.

John suggested at the meeting that the speech pathologist, physical therapist, occupational therapist, and nutritionist meet with the hospital rehabilitation team and jointly complete functional assessments. He suggested that the speech pathologist, occupational therapist, and nutritionist jointly evaluate Mrs. White's oral motor functioning and speech potential, and that the physical therapist and occupational therapist jointly evaluate mobility and use of limbs, nursing and occupational therapy would evaluate ADL skills, and the attending physician was to be included in all evaluations. John further suggested that the team presume Mrs. White would return to her apartment as the basis for care planning. The care plan would be developed at the next meeting.

Much to his dismay, the team members were reluctant to participate in the comprehensive geriatric assessment and team decision making format John was proposing. The members of the team were now openly being challenged to carry out the team reform proposal. After a period of unnerving silence, Louise Richards spoke. She said that, even if she and Ed McCarthy, the occupational therapist, could find time to make a joint visit to the rehabilitation hospital, or the nursing facility on Mrs. White's return, their disciplinary backgrounds would most likely result in divergent assessments. Although she felt there was considerable overlap between the disciplines, she believed there was sufficient difference to limit her understanding of the occupational therapy process, and vice versa. The discussion that followed indicated that most of the team felt joint evaluations were intuitively appealing, but impractical. Some team members felt they would spend too much time teaching other staff about their disciplines and not enough time doing the assessments. Although they agreed to attempt joint evaluations, most were skeptical as to their value.

John left the meeting disappointed and confused. He wondered what the outcome of the meeting would be as he sat looking over Mrs. White's medical reports. This case would require a concerted effort at rehabilitation to keep Mrs. White in her apartment in accord with her wishes. How could he get the team to see that the effort to return Mrs. White to independence required more than ordinary multidisciplinary information exchange? Even if he could convince the team, how could he convince Bill Wagner to support his position, given the financial implications?

To make matters worse, on his return from the meeting he found a note on his desk from Dr. Schmidt. The note read as follows:

> I am sorry I could not attend the meeting. I have spoken to Mr. Wagner and agree that Mrs. White cannot possibly continue to live in her apartment, despite her wishes. I have spoken to her daughter in St. Louis and she agrees it would not be safe for her mother to be on her own. I have therefore directed Mrs. White to be classified as a long-stay resident of the nursing facility and that her care plan include discharge to personal care when she has sufficient strength for mobility to go to the dining room. Please advise Mr. Wagner of this decision and let me know when Mrs. White will be discharged from the hospital.
>
> Aaron

Despite the reaction of the team and Dr. Schmidt's unilateral decision, John was committed to pursuing his team development strategy. He believed this was the only way to assure the continuous improvement in quality of services at GSV. Even if he lost the battle over Mrs. White's Care Plan, he would pursue these issues in other ways. Perhaps he had been too hasty in implementing a solution requiring team members to adopt behaviors with which they were unfamiliar and uncomfortable. John Evans had to wonder, what had gone wrong? What should he do now?

Lockwood Manor Convalescent Home: Admitting HIV/AIDS Residents to a Nursing Facility

Susan Lehrman

JENNY SCHRIVER, administrator of Lockwood Manor (LM) Convalescent Home, a 168-bed skilled nursing facility owned by a for-profit chain, is facing a major challenge: how to integrate HIV/AIDS residents into the facility with the least possible disruption. Jenny and her top administrative staff have sidestepped the issue of HIV/AIDS admissions for some time. Since LM historically has run at 97 percent occupancy, it has been relatively easy to claim a lack of beds—or inadequate expertise—when asked to take an HIV/AIDS patient. In reality, however, Jenny knows that their avoidance has been based as much on fear and general lack of preparation as on legitimate organizational limitations.

Jenny believes that avoidance of HIV/AIDS residents is no longer an option for LM. Until a few months ago, St. Catherine's Home for the Aged, a facility just up the street, had a dedicated HIV/AIDS unit and admitted the majority of residents needing long-term care in the area. Jenny and her staff found it relatively painless to turn away HIV/AIDS residents in good conscience, knowing they were welcome and could get excellent care there. Unfortunately, St. Catherine's recently closed its doors, leaving a large gap in the continuum of care for HIV/AIDS patients. Given the obvious need, pressure from hospital discharge planners who refer the majority of Lockwood's residents, rumblings from other

This case is loosely based on a number of case studies. Special thanks to Daniel Gentry and Toni Fogarty.

community organizations, and laws prohibiting discrimination against persons with HIV/AIDS, Jenny has decided that the facility can no longer evade this issue—they must begin to admit persons with HIV/AIDS. The decision is relatively clear, at least in Jenny's mind, but how to implement it is much less so.

Lockwood Manor is located in a medium-sized midwestern city with a growing HIV/AIDS population that lacks adequate services. A recent survey, conducted by a local AIDS activist group, not only highlighted the lack of long-term care services for AIDS residents, but also revealed a low level of knowledge about the disease in the community. According to the survey, reported in the local newspaper, misconceptions and prejudice abound.

Based on staff reactions to Jenny's hints that Lockwood might begin to take HIV/AIDS residents in the future, she is convinced that employee awareness of and attitudes toward HIV/AIDS are not much different from those of the community as a whole. Given the negative response of staff, she hasn't dared mention the possibility to residents or their families.

Unfortunately, it is not just frontline workers who appear resistant to the idea of serving HIV/AIDS residents. Lockwood's managers and the corporate headquarters' staff are not themselves in total agreement with Jenny's growing commitment to offering HIV/AIDS care.

The director of nursing, Sharon Jones, has pointed out that HIV/AIDS residents will likely need intensive and high technology services, like IVs and central lines, and will be on heavy medication regimens—care that is currently only available in Lockwood's 22-bed Medicare-certified wing. The staff, which works the facility's other 146 beds, lacks the skills necessary to service the subacute care needs of such residents. Sharon also pointed out that an AIDS activist group recently picketed a nursing home in a nearby state because they felt the facility was not providing adequate care. She is worried about similar problems arising at Lockwood.

The directors of a number of the other departments also seem resistant to serving HIV/AIDS residents. Jim Lange, the director of support services (laundry, maintenance, dietary, and housekeeping) is concerned about educating his ethnically diverse staff, many of whom do not speak English. The chief pharmacist, Cynthia Wong, is worried about management of the increased drug stock that would be needed by HIV/AIDS patients and the burden of participating in clinical drug trials. Joe O'Connel, the social worker, has indicated that increased staff will be needed to meet the special social needs of HIV/AIDS residents.

Corporate headquarters staff members have mixed feelings about Jenny's desire to admit HIV/AIDS residents. On the one hand, they are concerned that the provision of such care will be costly; on the other, if managed correctly, such a service could potentially be a money maker for the corporation. Further, they are worried about the facility's reputation in the community—some may be supportive of admitting HIV/AIDS residents as part of the home's mission, while others will fear and oppose these admissions.

Jenny needs to develop a strategy. She wonders what additional information to collect and how to deal with the many stakeholders interested in her decision.

12

The Commons: Adjusting to Relocation

Donna Lind Infeld

THE COMMONS was established in 1942 by a religious community in a midwestern city. It is a 180-bed facility with three distinct units of 60 beds each: Nursing (nonskilled care), Alzheimer's Care, and Skilled Care. Nine months ago it moved from its old site to a new 180-bed building located in the suburbs. The Commons had a reputation for being one of the best nursing homes in the area, but concerns about the quality of care have increasingly been expressed since the move. While the old building was always over 95 percent full, the new building still has not reached over 85 percent occupancy.

Organizational Structure and Management

The Commons has a large (45-member) Board of Directors. Over the past several years it has relied heavily on its executive director, Ken Esson, for operational information. As a result, most members of the board are not aware of what is currently happening.

The table of organization (Figure 12.1) shows a reporting structure involving the positions of medical director (Dr. Krall), director of nursing (Nancy Hurley), assistant administrator (Richard Reilly), and director of finance (Stan Lafond) as key executive positions reporting to the Mr. Esson.

As executive director of a large, nonprofit, religious nursing home, Mr. Esson has a wide range of responsibilities. In addition to being

This case is a composite based on consulting experiences at several nursing facilities.

Figure 12.1 The Commons Organization Chart

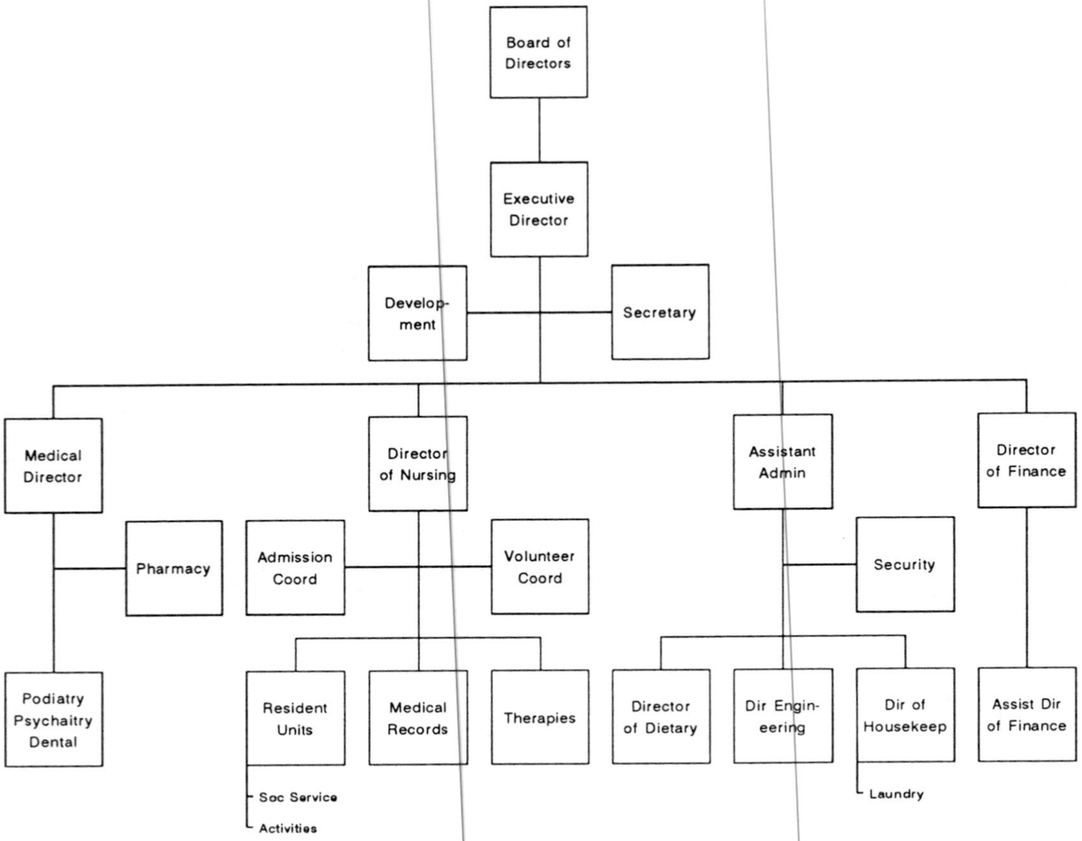

involved in day-to-day management, he is also the key link to the Board of Directors and is responsible for developing a long-term strategic vision for the Commons. Mr. Esson has been particularly busy with external matters since the move to the new building, but he is now becoming very concerned about internal developments. In the old building, things were running like clockwork, he thought. He asked the assistant administrator, Richard Reilly, to look into the situation and find out why things weren't going as smoothly now.

Richard was relatively new at the Commons, having been hired to plan and coordinate the move to the new facility. The move itself had gone quite smoothly. He currently is responsible for dietary, engineering, and housekeeping and laundry services. During his spare time over the next two weeks, Richard conducted interviews with staff, residents, and family members, as Mr. Esson had requested. At the top of his list of concerns were those related to quality of care:

- It took ten days of insisting on the part of a resident before she ever saw the doctor. Her incision was infected so she called her own doctor who sent a nurse over to pick her up. The Commons didn't even know she was gone. She has been rehospitalized, and the family doesn't want her readmitted here.
- A patient had a Stage II decubitus dressed on Friday. On Monday, the patient had the same bandage and the decubitus was Stage III. According to a nurse, "we just stumble onto problems because often they are not in the chart."
- A family member reported that a resident had bladder problems for eight to ten days before anyone suggested starting bladder training.
- A family member reported a period of overmedication and had to fight with staff to have it changed.
- A staff member told of a patient who usually could walk, and now was dragging her foot. After taking off her shoe the staff person noticed a large corn that should have been identified at a much earlier stage. Then the employee noticed numerous residents with broken toenails, commenting, "Little by little more residents with foot problems are not being reported to the podiatrist."

Medical Services

These complaints were surprising because the facility has an on-site medical clinic designed to provide the necessary care for skilled level patients. The home's medical director, Dr. Krall, is responsible for all physician services, with minimal private physician backup. However, a qualified and highly regarded physician assistant recently resigned, and Dr. Krall has been complaining about the need for more assistance.

Nursing Services

Nursing Services are organized into three resident care units: Nursing, Alzheimer's Care, and Skilled Care, each with its own unit director reporting to the director of nursing, Nancy Hurley. Social workers and activities staff have offices on each unit as part of the team approach to care, but they report to the director of psychosocial services. The former director of nursing resigned before the recent move because she didn't want to commute this far. Ms. Hurley, formerly a nurse at the Commons, was selected without a thorough search or the support of the medical director. She and Dr. Krall have different philosophies of care.

The team care approach is well-suited for the design of the new facility and the current nursing administration organization. While staff generally supports this approach, the home regularly experiences staff shortages and insufficient numbers of qualified nursing supervisors. While staffing levels are above legal requirements, extensive use of agency personnel has been necessary lately. For example, on a recent night shift, staffing included one RN, three LPNs, and nine certified nursing assistants (CNAs). Six of the CNAs were agency staff, unfamiliar with the residents, layout, and procedures of the Commons. Between 30 and 45 CNAs were hired from agencies in a recent two-and-one-half day period at twice the cost of staff CNAs.

Ms. Hurley has good clinical skills, but she does not possess the management competence required for her position. She spends most of her time in meetings with licensed nursing personnel instead of having a presence on the units with residents.

A particular problem is the functioning of the skilled unit. There are serious concerns about the unit director's clinical and supervisory skills. Nursing staff members on her unit were quick to offer examples of her inability to assist them in treating residents. Nursing staff reluctantly accepts assignment to the unit because of inadequate staffing for the heavy care needs of its residents. Similar concerns about staffing levels exist on the Nursing Care and Alzheimer's Care units.

CNAs were especially open with complaints, including low wages, poor benefits, and unfair treatment. There has been substantial turnover among CNAs recently. Of those hired in the last year, 32 percent of CNAs on the nursing unit, 35 percent on the Alzheimer's unit, and 65 percent on the skilled care unit have left.

Despite these problems, recent state surveys have not found many deficiencies in nursing services. Results of their most recent visit reported that:

1. No residents were receiving bowel and bladder training, and bowel and bladder evaluations had not been conducted on any of the incontinent residents.
2. In-service training sessions were inadequately attended by nursing staff. For most of the mandatory in-service sessions held last year, fewer than 20 percent of nursing staff attended.
3. Inspectors observed a medication pass with a 12 percent error rate. Errors included administering medication after meals when the order called for before meals and failure to administer drugs at the prescribed time in other instances.

Quality Assurance and Medical Records

Janet Robb is responsible for quality assurance and medical records, and she reports to the director of nursing, Ms. Hurley. While Ms. Robb told Mr. Reilly she didn't think things were really any different than in the old facility, nursing staff reported incomplete and inconsistent care plans and progress notes.

The most recent state survey findings indicated the following:

- Although separate care plans had been developed with ongoing goals and evaluations by the various professional services, inadequate verbal communication was occurring at daily administrative staff meetings regarding resident's problems and needs.
- The written resident's care plan was not comprehensive or interdisciplinary in content. All pertinent and active problems and needs were not identified, with input interventions from each discipline when appropriate.
- Care plans did not reflect that a coordinated and integrated plan of care was in effect for use by all resident care providers.

Although the survey team did not notice it, many members of the staff are concerned that during the month following the move to the new facility, nine deaths occurred (Table 12.1). Five of the nine deaths were on the Alzheimer's Care Unit, not on the Skilled Unit, where more would be expected.

Admissions

Vicki Wilkinson, a longtime employee of the Commons, is responsible for admissions, discharges, and transfers. She also reports to Nancy Hurley. Ms. Wilkinson is pressured to admit as many new residents as possible, given the recent declining census. Some nursing staff members have complained that when a new resident is admitted, information relating

Table 12.1 The Commons, Number of Deaths per Month

January	2
February	4
March	2
April	5
May	2
June	2
July	3
August	2
September	9
October	7
November	5
December	5

to his or her needs and medications is, on occasion, not efficiently communicated to the nursing unit.

Psychosocial Services

Social Services

This department is staffed with three full-time social workers, and three or more social work interns from the local university spend ten hours per week providing services to residents. The department manager aggressively locates less restrictive alternatives for residents who do not need nursing care. Since the social workers have offices on the units, they have excellent contact with residents, and nurses often turn to them for support.

Activities

The Activities program is designed to keep residents busy from morning until night. Staff constantly introduces new activities, but since the move to the new building, participation has fallen. The most recent state survey found that Social Services and Activities did not state measurable goals and specific approaches to the residents' problems in their records.

Moving to the new location has substantially increased the number of volunteers participating in activities at the Commons, because many members of the religious group live in nearby communities. As a result, activities staff has had to find new ways to keep them involved besides transporting residents to and from scheduled programs.

Food Service

Food service at the Commons is a major concern. While the food service manager appears to have the necessary skills and experience to direct the department, she is having problems because the new kitchen was poorly designed. It is crowded, has limited storage space, and has no serving line to set up meals quickly. She is angry that she was not consulted when the kitchen layout was being designed.

Residents are extremely dissatisfied with the quality and selection of food. There are constant complaints of cold, unappetizing food and unresponsiveness to individual requests and needs. The need for resident supervision and assistance during meal time also are frequent problems.

Employees complain about quality, selection, and long serving times. Food service employees are unhappy and express concerns about job security, wages, benefits, and transportation to work.

The most recent state survey reported some problems related to the delivery of nutrition to residents. For example, although medical records identified residents with low weight, poor nutritional intake, and unstable blood sugar levels, their goals and evaluations did not involve the dietary department. Surveyor observations of noon and evening meals revealed that once a food tray left the kitchen serving area, responsible disciplines were unable to determine if the portion size served was correct and, therefore, were unable to verify that the diet was served as ordered. For one patient with a fluid restriction there was no method to monitor the fluids that actually had been taken.

State surveyors also found unsanitary conditions in the food service area. Ice machines, a microwave oven, a cook's convection oven, a can opener, two vegetable freezers, and a baker's refrigerator needed cleaning. There was no thermometer in a vegetable freezer, and milk was leaking from cartons on the floor of the walk-in refrigerator.

Housekeeping and Laundry

The Housekeeping Department, while adequately staffed, is also experiencing management problems. The director of housekeeping has an ongoing conflict with her assistant, who sees herself as a co-director of the department. The housekeepers' loyalty and dedication to the residents has been undermined by this conflict. Poor wages, benefits, and unfair treatment also have contributed to recent employee dissatisfaction.

There appears to be adequate staffing, and acceptable services are provided by the laundry. Staff is very happy with its larger space and modern equipment at the new site. However, lost personal clothing continues to be reported.

Physical Plant and Maintenance

It is difficult to fully assess this department's ability to maintain the new building due to its short time of occupancy there. Staffing may need to be adjusted if the new facility's size and layout require additional attention.

The new building has an attractive, resident-focused layout. Unfortunately, program and living areas are far apart, and many residents need assistance to get around. Residents sometimes forego attending activities because of this, or else additional staff time is required to transport them.

The color scheme in the building is soothing and pleasing to the eye, but many residents have difficulty orienting themselves because it all looks alike. Carpeting in many heavily traveled hallways, while attractive, is difficult for residents to navigate, for staff to move various carts on, and for housekeeping to maintain. Another problem area for the engineering department is security. Better control of the flow of people and goods in and out of the facility is needed, especially in view of the large number of exits. Very few staff wear the required name badges.

With the Commons now located in the suburbs, the transportation needs of residents and staff are greater. Since the new facility is much farther from where most of the staff live, the Commons is offering a shuttle bus from the center of town. Staff members aren't happy with it, however, complaining that they have to leave home an hour earlier, and that the bus is crowded and uncomfortable.

Business Office

The Commons has an annual budget of approximately $8,500,000. Substantial private pay occupancy and charitable support are important factors in the financial picture of the home. The Business Office is headed by the director of finance and his assistant director. They are developing controls and accountability systems for the purchasing of goods and services. No established competitive purchasing procedure exists. Many employees have credit cards that are used to purchase items needed in their departments. The various staffs like this flexible aspect of the home's operations.

The Commons has one employee responsible for payroll and another responsible for personnel. They found this level of staffing to be necessary at the time of the move. The director of personnel is currently developing job descriptions and standards of performance for employees. Annual performance evaluations have not been conducted recently.

Many employees complained about salaries and wages. It is not clear, however, whether their wages really are below those earned in comparable positions in other facilities in the state (Tables 12.2 and 12.3). There also have been complaints by many staff members about their treatment by supervisory personnel.

Since Ken Esson was aware that staff might quit because of the location of the new building, he and the director of personnel developed a bonus program. A $50 bonus was awarded to all members of the nursing, dietary, and housekeeping staffs who stayed three months after the move,

Table 12.2 The Commons Salaries Compared to Salaries in Other State Nursing Homes

Salary	Low	High	Median	Mean	Commons
Admin.	$30,000	$145,000	$47,500	$60,400	$105,000
Asst. Admin.	31,200	57,200	37,600	46,750	52,000
DON	16,625	48,740	36,000	38,500	45,760

Typical Administrator Benefits Include:
• Medical insurance and hospitalization (33 percent require employee contribution averaging 1 percent of salary)
• Life insurance
• Dental insurance (56 percent covered)
• Disability (28 percent covered)
• A company car for 5 percent of administrators
• Average vacation time is 3.2 weeks/year with the average maximum accumulation of 4.5 weeks
• Retirement/pension plans provided to 67 percent of administrators; 42 percent must contribute to the plan
• Performance bonuses are received by 16.7 percent of administrators.

Table 12.3 The Commons Wages Compared to Wages in Other State Nursing Homes

Hourly Wage	Low	High	Median	Mean
RN—State	$10.80	$17.50	$12.35	$14.10
Commons RN	16.90	18.43	17.65	17.50
LPN—State	8.75	13.00	9.95	11.50
Commons LPN	9.95	13.92	11.95	12.30
CNA—State	5.20	7.30	6.20	7.05
Commons CNA	5.85	9.00	7.45	7.00

SOURCE: State Association of Homes for the Aging. Salary and Benefits Survey.

another $50 at six months, and a final $50 incentive was paid at nine months. They thought that after this much time most staff would be used to the new location. If some former staff did end up quitting, the bonus program was designed to help spread out termination dates and allow for new employees to be gradually hired from nearby neighborhoods. Unfortunately, the last bonus will be included with this month's paychecks, and there are rumors that widespread resignations will follow.

Resident Life

A large number of the residents who could communicate their feelings and experiences reported a strong degree of sadness and unhappiness about their new environment. A sample of their statements includes:

- This place is an institution; the old building was a home.
- This is a showplace for the ones who don't live here . . . for the ones who live here, it's hell.
- He doesn't give a damn for any of us. I hope when Mr. Esson gets old he has to take a bath in one of those bathers and sees how it feels.
- Management doesn't seem interested. We never see them on the floor.
- When I first came here, everyone was so friendly. I don't know why it changed.
- A lot of us are unhappy; I don't like what's going on.

Richard Reilly was overwhelmed. In addition to identifying the problems, he felt he should offer a plan to address them in his report to Ken Esson.

13

Holy Cross Medical Center/Transitional Care/Subacute Unit: Disaster Planning

Janet T. Reagan and Catherine Crowley

I awoke to a loud noise. I was scared to death! Knowing we were having an earthquake, I was sure my ventilator was going to bounce off the shelf and crash to the floor, disconnecting me from my life support system . . . and I would die. When the shaking finally stopped, the ventilator was still attached, and I was alive. Then the nurses came, they were calm and checked on me. They came around often and were very reassuring. The aftershocks were strong, and each one frightened me. I couldn't stop thinking that the next one would throw my ventilator to the floor.

The man who spoke these words is a quadriplegic who has spent the past 22 years on a ventilator. He suffered a loss of consciousness and an anoxic episode last year. He is frightened of many things now, but was terrified of the earthquake and aftershocks.

The Earthquake

At 4:31 a.m. on 17 January 1994, an earthquake measuring 6.8 on the Richter scale struck the San Fernando Valley area of greater Los Angeles. It was loud and powerful, wreaking havoc on the community. Residents of the area awoke to the violent shaking of their homes. Chimneys tumbled down, dishes became piles of rubble, furniture fell over, blocking exits,

This case is based in part on events that occurred at Holy Cross Medical Center, Mission Hills, California, during the 1994 Northridge earthquake that measured 6.8 on the Richter scale. Some events were fictionalized to enhance the case. Fictitious names were used for individuals throughout the case.

and the lights went out over most of Los Angeles. Common thoughts ran through the minds of all . . . Where are the children? Are they all right? Can I reach them? Where is the flashlight when I need it? How big is this quake, and what is the extent of the damage?

The "Northridge quake" caused a major disaster in Southern California. All of the health facilities in the San Fernando Valley sustained damage. Many were closed for days, and some for weeks.

The Medical Center

Located about two miles from the epicenter of the Northridge quake, this was the second largest earthquake to have struck the Medical Center in 20 years. The 1971 Sylmar earthquake badly damaged the Center's acute hospital, which was evacuated and rebuilt over the next few years with many joints reinforced beyond the code requirements of the day. These precautions probably resulted in the hospital's opening again just a week after the Northridge earthquake.

Holy Cross Medical Center's Transitional Care/Subacute Unit (TC/SAU) is adjacent to the main hospital campus. It was connected to the acute hospital by a tunnel that was rendered unusable by the Northridge quake. The one-story building was constructed in the sixties, originally serving as a rehabilitation unit, later as a skilled nursing unit, and even as an acute facility following the 1971 earthquake. On 17 January 1994, hospital patients were evacuated once again. Many were moved to the TC/SAU while they awaited transport to hospitals out of the area. Some remained in the unit until released to their homes.

The TC/SAU

The TC/SAU has 48 beds: 28 transitional care and 20 subacute. The Transitional Care Unit (TCU) is a high-acuity unit where patients spend from one day to a few weeks after acute hospitalization, receiving either rehabilitation therapies, medications, or both before moving to the next level of care, such as home or a skilled nursing facility. The patient mix is primarily geriatric. Patient acuity has increased markedly in the past two years. Oncology patients are cared for during radiation therapy; orthopedic and cerebral accident cases are also treated here. For most patients a primary focus is speech, physical, occupational, and respiratory therapies.

The Subacute Unit (SAU) was established one-and-a-half years ago as a long-term care, chronic ventilator dependent unit. The morning of the quake there were 16 ventilator-dependent tracheotomy patients on the unit and four patients who had tracheotomies only.

Impact of the Earthquake on the Hospital

The acute hospital sustained major damage. In the hospital staffing office, the night nurse supervisor was sitting at her desk across from the staffing clerk. Suddenly, the room was cast into complete darkness. She felt terrible shaking, and then a blow, as a large steel bookcase fell on her back. The staffing clerk was thrown across the room and realized that the supervisor was pinned under the bookcase. In an unusual show of strength, she pushed the bookcase away, freeing the supervisor.

Bruised and shaken, the nurse supervisor immediately began to assess the situation. If this was not the "Big One," it was certainly close. According to the Hospital Emergency Incident Command System (HEICS), she was in charge of the Medical Center until a higher ranking administrator arrived. Without lights and unable to locate a flashlight, she struggled into the hallway. The extensive damage left little doubt that she must activate Code Triage, the Disaster Plan for the Medical Center (Exhibit 13.1).

On the medical floors the patients were rudely awakened, plunged into total darkness, and terrified by the sounds of the earthquake. Televisions fell, IV poles tipped over, and the beds and consoles danced erratically around the rooms. When the shaking stopped, emergency lights could be detected in the hallways. Water ran here and there, and the dust was choking in some areas. Nurses began making rounds to check the condition of patients and to calm and reassure them. One by one, nurses began bringing patients into the hallways. They sat among the patients and talked reassuringly about the help that would soon arrive. Cracks in walls and stairwells were large, some ceiling tiles were down, and computer and telemetry monitors had fallen to the floor.

The critical care unit was busy as usual that night. When the first jolt came and lights went out, it took a minute for some of the nurses, who had been thrown across the room, to regain their bearings. Ventilators were off and nurses immediately began bagging (using a manual device for performing respiratory support) their patients until the emergency generator came on. They had only a split second in which to respond.

The nurse supervisor toured the facility, checking with head nurses on each unit. She knew all patients in the hospital would have to be evacuated, but did not know the extent of the damage in the community. Were they miles from the epicenter, and in better or worse shape than surrounding hospitals? Would they have to survive on their own for awhile or would help come, and how soon?

The CEO and chief engineer arrived at the Medical Center a little over an hour after the earthquake. Their survey of the facilities confirmed the nurse supervisor's assessment. All Medical Center buildings were

Exhibit 13.1 Policy/Procedure Medical Center and TC/SAU

Date Issued: 4/93   Title: Subacute Unit Disaster Plan
Date Reviewed:
Date Revised: Approved by: Safety Officer
Issued by: Subacute Unit   Date: 4/19/93

Purpose
To minimize loss of function, maximize available resources, and integrate into the Medical Center's overall Disaster Plan.

Policy
Each employee is responsible to know the Medical Center's Disaster Plan as well as their departmental plan and their role in it.

It is the responsibility of the Director of Clinical Services or his/her designee to inservice each employee at the time of department orientation and annually thereafter.

Procedure
Upon announcement of "Code Triage," the Director of Clinical Services or his/her designee will report to the auditorium or other announced location to be briefed on the following:

1. The nature of the disaster
2. The Medical Center's initial plan of action
3. The location of the EOC (Emergency Operation Center)
4. Told to report to the EOC for a possible assignment to the Hospital Emergency Command System
5. Told to initiate their department's Disaster Plan

Each Employee Will:
1. Check their area for injury to staff, patients, and visitors. Special attention should be paid to any patient on a ventilator

   Check:

   a. Ventilator is working properly; if not, ventilate patient with Ambu bag
   b. Oxygen is working properly; if not, switch to standby oxygen tank in the room. Then follow "Emergency Procedure for Isolated Hospitalwide Oxygen Pressure Failure"
   c. If ventilator is on battery power, plug ventilator into the red emergency power outlet in the hallway, using available extension cords.

   Note: The ventilator will only run 20 minutes to 45 minutes on battery power.
2. Check their area for damage
3. Assess their department's ability to perform in response to the disaster
4. Resource Nurse will assess the unit staffing needs and send available personnel to the Labor Pool in the construction trailer if not needed in the department

damaged, and the hospital had to be evacuated immediately. Aftershocks hit every few minutes; some were stronger than others. Would the next one cause the already weakened structures to collapse? The staff assumed that patients on the upper floors would have to be evacuated. How would they move 150 people from the third and fourth levels of the hospital? Staff members would have to carry them down the stairs, even though the stairwells were dim and shaking violently from aftershocks. They were aware of the extreme difficulty of functioning in a crisis and at personal risk, but they kept going. Their commitment to caring for the patients was tested that morning.

Fortunately, the TC/SAU fared better. It was decided to evacuate some patients to the TC/SAU. Arrangements were eventually made for others to be transferred to hospitals outside the affected zone. Staff needed to arrange an orderly evacuation and ensure that histories, medications, and transfer sheets accompanied patients.

The obstetrics unit was evacuated immediately. The critical care unit was evacuated separately, by helicopter and ambulances. Some patients from the Telemetry and Medical/Surgical units were discharged to their homes, and others were admitted to the TC/SAU sooner than expected. The hospital was closed; the only patients left at the Holy Cross Medical Center were on the TC/SAU.

Impact on Transitional Care/Subacute Unit

Patients transferred from the hospital were initially housed in the large TC/SAU dayroom, accompanied by their nurses from the Critical Care, Telemetry, Oncology, and Medical/Surgical units. Most patients remained calm and were cooperative. Staff from all units pulled together to ensure the well-being of patients. In several cases, physicians let their patients stay in the TC/SAU, rather than transfer them to another hospital, since they judged that the unit could continue to provide high-quality care. With the help of firemen and volunteers, all patients were evacuated from the acute hospital, and 18 hours after the earthquake, the last patient from the hospital was sent to the TC/SAU.

Ms. Jones, clinical manager of the unit, was at home when the earthquake hit. After recovering from the initial shock and finding her family safe, her immediate concern was for patients at the facility. The radio news reported that the epicenter was near Holy Cross Medical Center. Telephones were out. She had to get to the facility, but how? Would the roads be open? Freeways had collapsed during the 1971 quake; would they be safe now? Fortunately, the I-5 freeway was clear except for the crumbling walls along its sides. She interpreted the roller coaster feeling on the pavement as a sign to drive carefully.

TC/SAU Staff

That night, shift staffing for the TCU included one RN, one LVN, and three certified nurses aides (CNA). Staffing for the SAU consisted of two RNs, two licensed vocational nurses (LVNs), and four CNAs. When the quake hit, Ms. Lee, head nurse on the TCU, received a strong blow to the head. Stunned, but able to recover sufficiently, she helped check patients and directed the work of the rest of the staff. On the SAU, Ms. Thompson, the RN in charge, sustained a twisted ankle. Remaining staff members were shaken, bruised, and scared. They were worried about their patients and their families at home, yet, they carried on.

Until the clinical nurse manager arrived, Ms. Lee was responsible for the entire TC/SAU. She was thoroughly familiar with the Disaster Plan and had participated in two disaster drills, but she was stunned by the extent of the damage. Fearing aftershocks, Ms. Lee directed staff to check on the patients continually. She assessed the nature and seriousness of staff injuries, and was relieved to find that none was serious.

A Code Triage had been declared by the nurse supervisor, so Ms. Lee began to initiate the TC/SAU Disaster Plan. Satisfied with the safety of patients and staff, she began to assess the condition of the facility. It was difficult to move around. Furniture often blocked doorways, equipment, rooms, and hallways, and glass was everywhere. Ms. Lee directed two CNAs to begin clearing passages and cleaning up hazardous material.

Having survived the initial shock with only minor injuries, the patients and staff now faced another potential source of injury. The CNAs found their task difficult and sometimes impossible—where were the work gloves? Ms. Lee could not help; she knew work gloves and hardhats were essential, but did not know where they were stored. She suggested that they improvise—but not take unnecessary risks.

An LVN on the Subacute Unit asked Ms. Lee if she could leave to check on her family now that the patients had been checked and all appeared well. The LVN was the only registry staff on duty that evening, and this was only the second time she had worked at the Medical Center. Ms. Lee needed all the staff to stay, at least until some replacements arrived. She calmed the LVN, assigned her to work with an RN, and convinced her to remain until the day shift staff arrived.

Patients

Most patients fared well. None of the 14 patients on ventilators lost a breath; three backup systems were in place in the SAU. On the TCU, the patients also did well. Mr. Corona jumped out of bed and fell when the earthquake hit. A male nurse lifted him back onto the bed and, luckily, he was not seriously injured. Severely confused patients were particularly agitated and fearful. Ms. Kim insisted on leaving. Staff frequently assured her that when her family arrived she might be discharged. Ms. Atoyan insisted on sitting in the hallway for the first day-and-a-half. Seeing the activity of the staff seemed to have a reassuring and calming affect, and the staff were happy to accommodate her.

Emergency lights were dimmer than the normal lights, which troubled some patients, especially those with vision problems. All patients were anxious to learn about their loved ones and homes. Some patients were relieved to be in the TC/SAU, where they knew help was available, rather than at home alone.

The TC/SAU Facility

The facility withstood the initial shock and numerous aftershocks well. Although equipment, furniture, and supplies were thrown to the floor or shifted, there was no major structural damage. Patients did not have to be evacuated. The backup electrical system functioned immediately. Communication systems were down and the water supply was compromised, but these problems could be handled.

After the Earthquake

Ms. Jones, the clinical manager, arrived at the facility an hour after the initial shock. She immediately assessed the condition of the patients and staff. Ms. Lee had managed to function during the first hour after the earthquake, but her head injury was painful; with the arrival of Ms. Jones, she was relieved and sent home, as was the head nurse in the SAU. The condition of other staff and most patients appeared good, given the severity of the disaster. Disaster procedures were being followed and the facility was beginning to recover, just in time to come to the aid of the acute hospital.

Mr. Williams, CEO of Holy Cross Medical Center, informed Ms. Jones that patients had to be evacuated from the hospital to the TC/SAU. She would need to find space for as many patients as possible. In addition to overseeing the TC/SAU, she was put in charge of tracking nurses and hospital patients transferred to the TC/SAU.

The day shift was about to begin. Two RNs had already been sent home due to injuries, two CNAs and the LVN from the registry also went home. Although the injuries of the CNAs were not serious, they had families they felt they must attend to. Ms. Jones considered the remaining staff. How many could she count on to stay? How many of the day staff would be able to get to the facility?

Fortunately, most of the night staff stayed throughout the day. Some stayed up to 36 hours, even though they were worried about their families. Most day staff reported for work; however, some nurses could or would not come to relieve the night shift. Certain roads were impassable, and children could not be left alone because day care programs and schools were closed.

Most therapy had to be canceled or limited to bedside exercises due to the numerous aftershocks. One physician arrived within hours and discharged many of the rehabilitation patients. They were sent home with the assurance they could return for therapy when the aftershocks subsided.

Some families were able to get through to the facility. No calls could go out, but occasionally a call would be received. A few families simply arrived to check on a patient and take him or her home. Beds vacated by discharged rehabilitation patients were filled by patients evacuated from the hospital. Fortunately, some hospital staff remained to augment the unit staff and care for these patients.

Even though operating under extraordinary circumstances, patients received care. Communications, however, continued to be a problem, and available water was sporadic and not suitable for human consumption. Ms. Jones was able to get the bottled water company to commit for three times the normal order for as long as needed. Hand washing was never compromised due to the use of aseptic solutions throughout the facility. Electricity was not available for over two days, but the backup system did not falter. Even dietary was able to muddle through. The first meals were cold, but no meals were missed. On the second day, there was even a hot dinner for both patients and staff. Similarly, the pharmacy, laundry, housekeeping, and engineering departments were able to continue functioning despite the disaster.

Response to the Disaster

Three months after the Northridge quake, the Safety Officer and Safety Committee were directed to evaluate the adequacy of Holy Cross Medical Center and TC/SAU's response to the earthquake and to make recommendations for revising the Disaster Plan.

Recommended Readings

Joint Commission on the Accreditation of Health Care Organizations. 1993. *1994 Accreditation Manual for Long-Term Care, Volume 1: Standards.* Oakbrook Terrace, Illinois.

Federal Emergency Management Agency. National Emergency Training Center. 1989. *Nonstructural Earthquake Hazard Mitigation for Hospitals and Other Health Care Facilities.* Emmitsburg, MD: Emergency Management Institute.

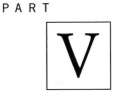
Human Resources and
Labor Relations

Chapel Square Health Care Center: Professional Diversification

Jeffrey A. Kramer

Background

CHAPEL SQUARE HEALTH Care Center, a skilled nursing facility, is one of a decreasing number of labor-intensive organizations continuing to operate in New Haven, Connecticut. Once a thriving New England city, New Haven has been hard hit by a middle class exodus to the suburbs, intense poverty, and rising crime rates. Chapel Square Health Care Center was built in an era when elderly people requiring institutional health care intentionally sought out care in New Haven. It was built in 1977, by John Stearns, a long-term care facilities developer who foresaw a need for long-term care beds in the heart of urban areas. In the 1970s he invested heavily in this and similar projects throughout the northeast. Chapel Square was one of nine facilities he built during this period, and one of the first to have become unionized.

Chapel Square originally had 180 beds, providing both skilled and intermediate care. From the late 1970s to the mid-1980s occupancy was quite high, typically close to full occupancy. To ensure this high census, Chapel Square expanded its patient base beyond geriatric patients to include mentally retarded and mentally ill patients transferred from state facilities. In these cases, the facility's primary mission of caring for the elderly was subverted for the sake of guaranteed reimbursement and filled

Fictitious names of both the organization and individuals are used to ensure anonymity.

beds. This strategy provided short-term profitability, but had long-term repercussions.

In the mid-1980s, Chapel Square experienced a significant decline in demand. The diversified resident population alienated geriatric patients from interest in the facility. Neighborhood decline had become noticeably worse, with crime and drugs more prevalent. In addition, a dwindling pool of private pay patients intensified competition from other facilities struggling to maintain high occupancy. Many adopted specialized services such as subacute care programs, Joint Commission on the Accreditation of Healthcare Organizations (JCAHO) facility accreditation, and other methods to distinguish themselves from their competitors. Further, the physical plant of the facility had deteriorated to the point where it affected the ability to recruit patients and staff, and jeopardized compliance with state and federal regulations.

Renovations

These problems became more pronounced in the late 1980s. Desperately trying to stay afloat, Chapel Square launched an ambitious construction program in the early 1990s. The project included renovation of the existing structure, improvement of the physical plant, and major expansion, adding 60 skilled nursing beds. The rationale was that additional beds in a new wing would enhance Chapel Square's failing reputation, attract more private pay residents, and introduce economies of scale. The original intermediate beds would be converted to skilled beds. While the risk associated with the project was considerable, it was viewed as a last resort for long-term survival of the facility. Renovations and construction of the new wing were completed three years ago.

Management

During this period facility ownership and management changed several times. While the facility remained proprietary, several owners had experimented with various management approaches at Chapel Square. During its history, the facility had been led by several well-intentioned, but variously effective, administrators, contract management services, and management teams. Shortly after the construction was completed a new administrator, Ketty Hansen, was hired to "turn things around."

Hansen was not discouraged by the problems Chapel Square presented. She had worked in a number of inner city facilities and was accustomed to the challenges of managing problem-plagued facilities. She was pleased by the physical plant improvements. Almost immediately she identified three major, interrelated problems needing attention if

Chapel Square was to survive and prosper: an exceptionally low private pay census, a poor reputation for quality, and a workforce characterized by a unionized staff and ethnic diversity that led to problems in this instance.

Low private pay census was common throughout the industry. Although nearly all of the mentally retarded and mentally ill patients had been transferred or discharged to other facilities, Chapel Square could not shake this reputation. It now housed a diverse resident population in terms of ethnic distribution, with a patient mix of approximately 30 percent Caucasian, 30 percent African American, 30 percent Hispanic, and 10 percent from other ethnic backgrounds. Even with new skilled beds in tastefully decorated units, the facility did not appeal to patients with financial means. As a result, Chapel Square was heavily dependent upon Medicaid reimbursement. With only 0.5 percent of the census private pay and five percent Medicare, approximately 94 percent of patients were supported by Medicaid. This was compounded by an overall census of about 70 percent occupancy, a lower level than was needed to reach reasonable profitability. Hansen viewed the less than full cost reimbursement from Medicaid and the low overall occupancy rate as pressing problems requiring immediate attention.

Hansen was also deeply concerned about Chapel Square's ongoing reputation for poor quality. Its inner city setting did not help the situation, and the many survey deficiencies the facility had received over the years only made a bad situation worse. While candidly admitting to herself and a few others that it was deserved, Hansen recognized that measures were needed to reverse these impressions.

When Hansen was offered the administrator's position, she knew that Chapel Square was unionized and had a diverse workforce. Having worked in unionized facilities before and established a good rapport with union leaders, she had earned a reputation for managing human resources successfully. However, she quickly discovered an unprecedented level of dysfunctional behavior among the Chapel Square staff. She set to work to address these problems.

Management Problems

Hansen observed a number of existing behavioral and facility management problems contributing to the poor quality of care. Basic supplies were lacking to the point where care was compromised. The facility was so short of bed linen that it was used until it literally fell apart. The prevailing attitude by staff about supplies was, "We're not going to get them, so why bother even asking."

There was a desperate need to change ingrained behaviors and philosophies. Historically, employees felt abused by management, and a sense of complacency had resulted. Chapel Square had become a facility without a spirit. Staff's complacency about quality of the care contributed to even poorer conditions. Having faced decertification on several occasions, deficiencies and citations had become a regular part of doing business. Hansen was appalled that the facility was dirty and that the nursing staff was poorly trained and not capable of meeting patients' nursing needs. Verbal abuse of residents by staff was a regular occurrence. The dietary department used only two menus, alternated weekly. Overall, the facility was locked into a pattern of poor quality care that had become the norm and was quickly adopted by newly hired staff.

Unionized positions at Chapel Square typically paid three to four dollars more per hour than at other facilities, helping ensure a steady flow of job applicants. The facility had agreed in past negotiations to these union demands to avoid a lengthy and damaging strike. These salary levels raised costs, but did not seem to improve performance.

Hansen saw the staff as a dysfunctional family, with communication barriers resulting from ethnic and cultural differences. New staff often came from the ethnic networks of current Chapel Square staff. Many workers were members of large extended families that had immigrated to the United States in recent years. While this made for easy recruitment, it also tended to divide staff along ethnic lines. Intra-staff communication was essentially nonexistent. Hansen viewed this as a problem needing a solution if she was to succeed in improving patient care services.

The Workforce

Chapel Square's staff reflects the "melting pot of America." It is dominated by three major immigrant groups: West Indians, Hispanics, and Indians from Southern Asia. West Indians are the largest group, representing 50 percent of the registered nursing staff, the majority of nursing management, 50 percent of the housekeeping department, 75 percent of certified nursing assistants (CNAs), and the entire dietary department. They primarily are from Jamaica and Haiti. Members of the Hispanic group come mainly from Cuba, Puerto Rico, and Costa Rica. They, too, represent a significant proportion of the overall staff.

Thirty-five percent of registered nurses, 24 percent of CNAs, 50 percent of housekeeping staff, and the entire maintenance staff are from Hispanic regions. The third largest group, the East Indians, are spread throughout the facility without large representation in any given department. Other ethnic and national groups adding to the diversified workforce consist of Africans, Caucasians, African Americans, and Chinese, respectively.

During her first few months at Chapel Square, Hansen observed differing behavioral patterns between the groups, including different levels of education, cultural values, participation in facility management, and communication styles. The large ethnic groups tended to have hierarchical structures reinforcing differences among the nationalities. For example, among West Indians, a class system seemed to exist, which placed Jamaicans above Haitians and other West Indians. The Hispanic hierarchy tended to value Cuban workers over Costa Ricans and Puerto Ricans. East Indians lacked a hierarchical structure; a characteristic Hansen found of interest given the rigid caste system in that country. However, East Indians were often the most distant group, rarely interacting with other nationalities in the work setting.

Varying levels of education also seemed to strain relationships. Jamaicans and Africans were typically the most highly educated. It was not unusual for these CNAs to hold masters degrees, since recent immigrants were often unable to secure other jobs. Hispanics usually had less formal education, and this often strained relationships with other staff. Caucasians and Indians were usually well-educated, although this varied considerably.

To a large extent, Chapel Square's management team reflected this melting pot of nationalities, although it was overly represented by Caucasians. The administrator, Hansen, and her assistant administrator, Bob Manning, were Caucasian, as were all of Chapel Square's department heads. For example, while the entire dietary staff was Jamaican, the dietary department head was Caucasian, and the assistant department head was Hispanic. Among the other assistant department heads there was one other Hispanic and one Caucasian. Of 13 nursing department managers there were six West Indians, one African, and two African Americans. The nursing staff, while not part of management, was truly a mix of nationalities: 50 percent West Indian, 35 percent Hispanic, and the remaining 15 percent Caucasian or Chinese.

Hansen recognized that cultural, religious, educational, language, and economic differences among the various nationalities that composed the Chapel Square staff were affecting patient care and facility management. Communication problems were widespread, and little was being done to resolve the confusion they created. For example, Jamaican CNAs would talk to Jamaican nurses, but not to Hispanic nurses. Most West Indians, Hispanics, and Indians would not communicate with African nurses. In general, the staff did not seem to communicate well with either their superiors or their subordinates. Communication linkages were further strained by each group's preference to communicate in their native language, even if they knew English.

Hansen realized that it was necessary to try to change old behaviors and philosophies. She began by replacing some existing department heads, appointing ones she felt would be more supportive of this effort. Until that time, line staff had not been given a lot of direction. She also identified informal leaders among the staff, representing various ethnic groups, to help work on the communication problems. These leaders served as interpreters during meetings and tried to help overcome cultural barriers. They understood the need for change, and served an important role in facilitating the process. While this approach was marginally effective, the unevenness of the leaders' dedication to the proposed changes limited its impact.

Other approaches were also used to improve communication within the facility. Small-group in-service training programs were developed by the administrative staff to promote attitudinal changes. Outside consultants were brought in with packaged training programs to improve staff communication, but their failure to address the needs of the diversified workforce at Chapel Square led to disappointing results. Hansen also began to emphasize an informal management style that took into account the unique characteristics of the facility. She spoke frequently of a team orientation and spent considerable time with management staff reinforcing concepts of team building and group consensus.

Management's Dilemma

Despite these efforts, there was little progress toward improved communication. Hansen and the management team, which consisted of Manning and all of Chapel Square's department heads, became increasingly convinced that the communication problems that led to inconsistent patient care were more a result of cultural differences than anything else. Hansen noticed that not all groups were equally receptive to the changes being implemented. East Indians accepted the process without much resistance. Hispanics and Haitians, who had the least developed English skills, were not as responsive, and posed a more difficult challenge.

Two years ago, after several frustrating months of trying to improve internal communication, Hansen formed a Cultural Awareness Committee. The committee was comprised of representatives from all major groups in the facility. Special attention was given to selecting members who were both respected by their fellow workers and had demonstrated willingness to improve the facility's patient care and overall performance. The committee was given a charge by Hansen to develop activities for the staff to minimize the effect of cultural differences, while lowering barriers to change.

Occupancy had remained relatively constant at 70 percent, and the facility seemed unable to shed its "poor quality" reputation. To improve quality of care, Hansen and Manning were convinced they needed to improve communication and bring about facilitywide behavioral changes. Otherwise, Chapel Square would continue to lose market share in an increasingly competitive marketplace. The corporate offices, while supportive of the management team at Chapel Square, were also losing patience. Without improvements in the financial situation through a higher patient census, the possibility of the facility being sold or declaring bankruptcy could not be ruled out.

Hansen worked with the Cultural Awareness Committee during the next few weeks to help participants develop their agenda. She reinforced the notion that the committee should plan activities whereby "each group could be proud of its own culture, but understand other cultures." The first idea that surfaced was for a mini-exhibition including exhibits from each cultural group. However, this idea was rejected because many committee members felt it would lead to further isolation, rather than facilitating communication and consensus. Finally, in January, the committee endorsed the idea of a Cultural Day to include costumes and foods from the many ethnic and cultural groups. While not significantly different from the first idea, the committee was enthusiastic. Although somewhat skeptical, Hansen threw her support behind the idea and met with the committee to assist with their preparations.

As Cultural Day approached, Hansen continued to work on several different fronts. She met regularly with the Cultural Awareness Committee and made sure they had ongoing input and support from the management team. She visited each patient care unit almost daily, getting to better know and understand the staff, residents, and families. Concurrently, she met informally with many members of the staff to solicit their opinions about how to improve the facility and its image.

On a separate track, Bob Manning was assigned to monitor Chapel Square's adherence to health regulations. He responded with a "certification watch" which simulated the inspection process. Finally, realizing that additional steps were needed, Hansen called together her management team. She asked them to begin work on a long-term strategic plan to improve communication among the facility's ethnic and cultural groups. It was hoped that this would lead to improvements in patient care. A draft document outlining their ideas was to be submitted to her for initial review. They began to work on this arduous task the following day, aware of the many obstacles facing them.

Jennett Manor: Employee Complaints

Alice L. O'Neill

Introduction

JENNETT MANOR, a 120-bed proprietary long-term care facility, is located in Dunham, a small New England town. Area residents tend to have a solid work ethic and strong family ties. Community and family members visit the facility regularly, often assisting with meals and activities.

Jennett is the primary local employer; the other is a garment factory. There are two other long-term care facilities and two acute care facilities within 20 miles. The facility was built 15 years ago to meet the growing need for skilled nursing facilities (SNFs) and intermediate care facilities (ICFs). There are 60 skilled beds and 60 intermediate care beds at Jennett Manor; 10 additional ICF beds are being planned for.

Neither Jennett nor the local garment factory are unionized, however, Local 1199, of the Service Employees International Union (SEIU), and the state nurses' association represent employees at the two nearby acute care facilities.

Four weeks ago, the administrator, James Boland, submitted his letter of resignation to the board of directors. He wanted to move closer to his family in the Midwest and was actively seeking employment there.

The Board of Directors

The four members of the board are also the owners of Jennett Manor. Although none of the board members has health care–related experience,

This case is based on a real organization, but names of people and places have been changed to assure anonymity.

Figure 15.1 Jennett Manor Organization Chart

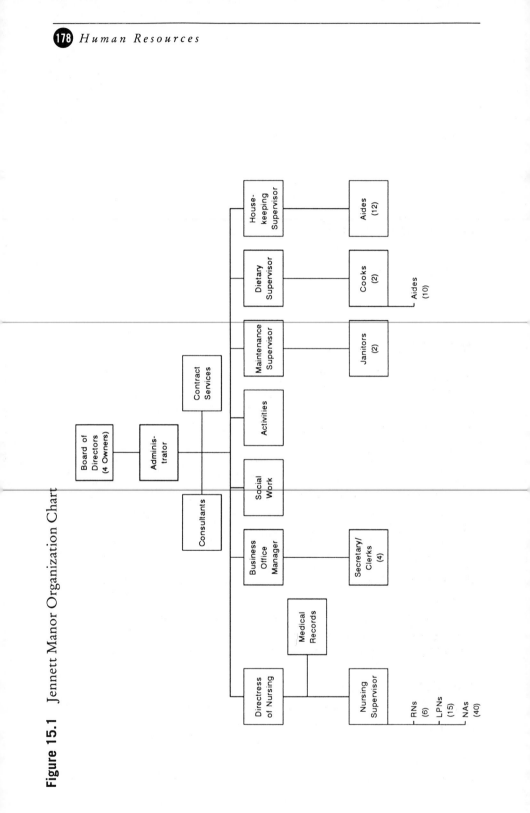

each has a successful private business. Only one of the owners lives in Dunham, and none of their businesses are unionized. The board meets monthly and the administrator and the business manager attend each meeting. Following its search, the board recruited and hired Maureen MacDonald.

Jennett's Employees

The organization of the 100-person staff at Jennett Manor is depicted in Figure 15.1. Most nonprofessional employees live in or near Dunham. It has always been difficult for Jennett to recruit and retain RNs. Although it is easier to recruit nursing assistants, once trained, many leave to be employed at a local hospital within six months of being hired. Jennett provides employee benefits to full-time personnel, who may also purchase coverage for a spouse or family members through the facility's plan.

In addition to regular staff, Jennett contracts for the services of a registered dietician, a registered records analyst, and a certified recreation activities therapist. Physical, occupational, and speech therapies, as well as pharmacy, dental, radiology, laboratory, laundry, and medical director's services are contracted locally. Nursing staff are often obtained from a professional pool agency to cover staff shortages.

Residents

Admission to Jennett Manor has been competitive, with a 98 percent occupancy rate. There is usually a waiting list of potential residents from nearby and outlying hospitals. While most residents are admitted with Medicare coverage, they frequently revert to medical assistance after lengthy stays. The average length of stay is two years. About 15 percent have private insurance, 7 percent are private pay, and a few are covered by veterans benefits. Seventy percent of residents are female, with an average resident age of 74 years. Primary diagnoses of Jennett's residents are: stroke, hip fracture, congestive heart failure, diabetes, chronic obstructive pulmonary disease, chronic organic brain syndrome, skin ulcers, and Alzheimer's disease.

The Situation

James Boland had given the board six weeks of notice, but it was not until three weeks before he was due to leave that Maureen MacDonald was contacted. Maureen had been assistant administrator at Fairway Acres, a 90-bed skilled nursing facility, for three years. Although it was a unionized facility, labor-management relations were amicable. Maureen believed that employees intend to do a good job and, with management support, they will "give 100 percent." She was respected at Fairway Acres because she treated employees fairly.

Fairway's administrator supported Maureen's decision to interview at Jennett Manor. Maureen had planned and implemented some excellent programs at Fairway (both employee–oriented and community relations–oriented), and he felt Maureen could bring a lot of expertise to Jennett Manor.

During the interview, the board proudly reported no significant negative comments from the Department of Health (DOH) in recent surveys. The board was very complimentary about the "tight way" the director of nursing (DON), who had been at Jennett for eight years, and the nursing supervisor, who had been there for six years, "ran the ship." In fact, it was due to their efforts that the facility had avoided a sit-down strike and possibly a unionization attempt by nursing assistants. The board believed a big problem was with the recruitment of RNs and LPNs; they just didn't like to work in nursing homes.

Maureen decided to accept the position and resigned from Fairway Acres, giving four weeks notice. During this time, in accordance with the recommendation of the Jennett board, she contacted Mr. Boland. Unfortunately, he was unable to meet with her because he was busy preparing for his move. He invited Maureen to visit the facility and use his office to review records. Maureen understood his situation.

A Visit to Jennett Manor

Maureen was greeted by a secretary and several department heads who stopped by during her visit. Unfortunately, the DON and the nursing supervisor were away at a seminar. As she reviewed the facility's policies and procedures, Maureen noted that several required updating to meet licensure regulations. She decided this would be a priority for the first department head meeting. At the end of the day she was given a tour of the facility.

Following this visit, Maureen telephoned Mr. Boland. He said that anything else she needed she could get from the DON and the nursing supervisor. He was leaving a week earlier than expected to interview for an new position.

The Job Begins

On Maureen's first day at the job, she received a "welcome" bouquet of flowers from the department heads. The DON and the nursing supervisor were on vacations granted by Mr. Boland and not returning for another week. Over the next week, Maureen visited every resident, met with each department head, and greeted employees individually. Family members and those residents who were able stopped in to wish her good luck.

Maureen was very concerned about several documents unavailable for review and others seriously needing to be updated. The missing information was supposed to be on Mr. Boland's computer, but it could not be found. It was impossible to contact him since he did not leave a forwarding address or telephone number.

Several employee personnel files lacked current performance evaluations, mandated health records, and evidence of orientation to the facility. Maureen also noted that previously, on two consecutive DOH survey visits, recommendations had been made to improve nursing documentation and nursing department management procedures. The high turnover rate in the nursing department that had been mentioned by the board was clearly in evidence.

Jennett did not have a wage and benefit policy; personnel were hired and quoted a starting wage by department heads using their own judgement. Personnel, especially in the nursing department, received wages much below those of competitor facilities. Significant overtime was paid to a few nursing employees.

Maureen decided that she would meet with the DON to discuss employee records and the wage policy. Then they could develop policies for board approval. A cursory review of resident medical records revealed that the mandatory monthly charting was not up-to-date, however residents appeared to be well taken care of and families had not complained. Maureen was surprised the facility had not received more survey deficiencies from the Department of Health (DOH). Several areas needed prompt attention and she hoped to get them cleared up prior to the expected "new administrator survey" the DOH always performed.

The next Monday, the DON and the nursing supervisor returned to work. They mentioned a close relationship with Mr. Boland and hoped for the same with Maureen. He "pretty much allowed them to run the building, and things had gone smoothly." There were, however, a few times when it had not been so smooth, like when evening shift NAs threatened a "sit-down." The nursing supervisor had returned from home and told them they could lose their jobs if they did not get back to work. There had been no problems since then.

They mentioned a few really dedicated NAs. Some, especially the many single parent heads of households, needed the money and would always accept overtime. Others would call in sick and then be seen shopping on Main Street. In addition, two RNs, out on Worker's Compensation, were really malingerers, and the facility would be better off without them.

Maureen asked about the files she was looking for but they could offer no help. She also asked them to get Mr. Boland's address or phone number if he contacted them. Finally, she asked them to develop a plan to get the charting done as quickly as possible, before the DOH held a surprise survey.

Next, Maureen met with the business manager, whom she asked to conduct a wage and benefit survey of area long-term care facilities and hospitals, in preparation for a standardized salary structure proposal to the board.

A few days later the nursing supervisor told Maureen she and the DON were scheduled to attend another seminar the next day; Mr. Boland had approved it. At 10 a.m. that day, Maureen answered a knock on her office door. Five NAs wanted to talk to her privately. They asked her to keep their comments confidential because they were all afraid of losing their jobs. They complained that the DON and the nursing supervisor played favorites. Poor performance evaluations and last minute schedule changes resulted if they protested. "They can make our lives miserable if they find out about this meeting and I really need this job," one said. Another asked, "Why do you think so many NAs leave? It's because we're treated so terrible by the nursing supervisor, and the DON just backs her up." They told Maureen to "Ask Mr. Jones' (a resident) wife how the nursing supervisor treats us." They hoped she would not be taken in like Mr. Boland was; they heard from NAs at Fairway Acres that Maureen was a fair person. By the way, did Maureen know, they asked, that Mr. Boland had called the DON and the nursing supervisor at the facility several times since leaving Dunham? Needless to say, Maureen was very surprised.

Now she was really in a quandary. Did the NAs have a basis for their complaints, or was it just "sour grapes" because they had been reprimanded by the DON or the nursing supervisor? She resolved to get to the bottom of this.

When Maureen drove into Jennett Manor the next morning, she saw union organizers passing out leaflets near the facility entrance. Maureen was worried about the pending DOH survey; she did not need this new problem right now. Things were clearly not as they had seemed when she interviewed for the position at Jennett Manor.

Westview Nursing Home: Labor Relations in a Unionized Nursing Facility

Jan M. Fritz

SHE COULD see the Terminal Tower in the pre-dawn darkness as the Cleveland bus carved its way through the downtown area, heading for the near West Side. Hattie Green still found it an impressive building, even if it was no longer the city's tallest, but the other passengers didn't even look out the windows and some appeared to be napping. There had been few riders on the bus at 5:30 a.m. when she had boarded on the East Side, but there always were more on this second bus, the one she caught downtown. Hattie, a 52-year-old African American woman, had been a nursing assistant on the first shift at the Westview Nursing Home for more than 15 years, so she knew most of the other early morning travelers by sight, if not by name.

This morning, November 1, would be the first day of contract negotiations, an event that happened every three years. The contract renewal date at Westview is December 20. Hattie again would be part of the negotiating team, and looked forward to getting the work behind her.

Hattie recalled how twenty years ago she and a friend went to two informational meetings of 1233, a union. They came back convinced that it was important to get the other workers to fill out union cards and work as a group to bargain for benefits, better wages, and a voice for employee rights.

The facility, including its characters and events, are fictitious. They are based on professional experience and extensive interviews by the author.

The author wishes to thank her assistant, Brian Martens; arbitrators; and labor union officials for their help. The author particularly wishes to acknowledge the key contributions of many nursing homes, administrators, unionized employees, ombudspersons, owners, and union organizers.

Hattie had gone to the nursing home's office only one week before the first 1233 meeting to learn about purchasing health insurance. She had two small children then and wanted the security of having insurance. The woman behind the desk told Hattie she didn't make enough money to even consider buying insurance. Hattie really liked her job, even if the wages weren't very good, but she knew she would have to do something about getting her family health insurance.

Every time the union contract came up for renewal, Hattie couldn't help but think about the earliest contract negotiation periods. Some had been very difficult; the first ones had been the worst. Management had been arrogant, dragged out the many meetings over six-month periods, delayed signing the contracts, and made life in general very hard.

Things were much different now. For instance, negotiation meetings for many years were held in hotel conference rooms, as there was a lot of concern about neutral turf. The last contract discussions were held in the office of management's lawyer because the union agreed that it was convenient and that there was a continuing, productive relationship between the two sides.

The Westview Nursing Home is located on West 25th Street, just past the open-air West Side Market. The market opens early and Hattie watched the vendors putting out their vegetables and fruits as the bus pulled up to the home.

• • •

Connie Thomas, an African American 22-year-old, has worked as a nursing assistant at Westview for nine months. Her mother and father worked hard to give their daughters opportunities they hadn't had and encouraged them to go on to school. Her mother always said, "You will never lose if you have the training to be a nurse." Connie took the nursing aide job to help pay for her education. She is studying to be a registered nurse.

Connie parked her car on a side street and raced for the time clock to punch in by 7 a.m. She had been reprimanded once for being late, and knew that if she punched in more than ten minutes early or late she would have to get her time card approved by the supervisor. She "didn't want to be discussing punctuality again," so she was really moving when she met up with Hattie.

Hattie reminded her that the union caucus before the first negotiation session would begin promptly at 4:30 p.m. and, as Connie had never been through this, she should make sure to be on time. Hattie told her not to worry about dinner because there would be some food available in the negotiating room.

Connie's older sister had worked "in dietary" and convinced her to take the job at Westview even though she had to travel from the East

Side. She wasn't sure she liked it. Probably her biggest concern was that she hadn't realized how hard the job was going to be.

Connie had to get four people up, washed, groomed, and dressed and see that they got to breakfast in a little over an hour each morning. Connie could get Mr. Jesensky ready quickly, but Miss Kossuth's mind was completely gone, as Connie told her friends, and Miss Kossuth was difficult. Miss Kossuth always "had four or five layers of clothing on" and they had to be removed before Connie could even get started. Then there was Mr. Kundtz, who was verbally abusive and never wanted to get out of bed, and Miss Petrash who would only eat breakfast if Connie stayed with her.

Connie delivered meals to the four other people on her floor because they couldn't come down for breakfast. Two had to be fed and one had to be assisted with her breakfast. After Connie straightened all the rooms and returned the breakfast trays, she could start on the showers and baths.

Each person got a shower or bath at least twice a week and Connie needed to change the bed sheets after helping them. This morning she was scheduled to give three showers, and she had barely finished before it was time to get "her people" to lunch. She took Mr. Jesensky down in his wheelchair, but she had to do Miss Petrash's make-up and hair (again) before she would go to lunch. (The nursing aides thought Miss Petrash was vain, but that she was "a pretty little thing and always wanted to look just right.") Miss Kossuth's private aide had arrived by now, which would make things go a little faster. Connie got her four people to lunch and delivered four meals to the others in their rooms.

After returning the lunch trays, Connie had time to help another aide with two patients who were too heavy for one person to assist alone. Then Connie had to cover another floor for the staff who wanted to go to lunch. Connie usually got a 15-minute break in the morning, but today she had been on her feet for five hours without a break and was looking forward to her own lunch.

• • •

Julia Zrencsik—white, 26 years old and single—had welcomed the opportunity to take the assistant administrator position at Westview. After receiving her graduate degree in gerontology, she went to work for a national nursing home chain for a little over one year. It had been a good experience, but she wanted to work in her hometown and in an organization where she would spend more time with residents and staff and a little less time on business concerns. When she was offered the job at Westview, she jumped at the chance.

Julia grew up in a suburb of Cleveland, but her Hungarian-American grandmother had been born in this neighborhood. While Julia didn't know any of the home's residents before coming here, she was somewhat familiar with the Hungarian culture shared by most of them. She also knew their neighborhood parish, St. Elizabeth, where one mass each week was still conducted in Hungarian, even though the neighborhood now included yuppies (young urban professionals), Appalachian white families, a multitude of Hispanic families, and a diminishing number of elderly, single Hungarians.

Julia did not feel prepared to work in a unionized facility and this would be her first contract negotiation. No one in her family had ever been a union member and the only discussion about unions she recalled was with an uncle, a comptroller for a large chemical company. He was opposed to unions because he thought they were difficult to deal with, corrupt, and frequently acted like "thugs" in trying to make things go their way. Besides that, he had said, they were dying out.

Julia's personnel courses at the university had dealt with management issues regarding workers, but included no labor history, and, she admitted to her friends, she had a hard time sorting out all the different unions and their relationships. Some of Julia's professional magazines included articles about "minimizing the union threat," and her previous employer had paid for her to attend a workshop on preventing unionization in a health facility. Yet Westview's management didn't seem to really mind the union, and Julia had grown to have a lot of respect for Hattie Green, the union's representative. Hattie seemed to get along very well with the other workers in the nursing, dietary, housekeeping, laundry, and maintenance departments, the areas represented by the union.

During Julia's first month at Westview, the owners had to deal with a family emergency, and Hattie was one of those asked to assist Julia. Julia learned that Hattie was genuinely concerned about the well-being of the residents, but was also deeply committed to her union and the well-being of union members. Julia knew Hattie had been elected to represent the home on the union's three-state, regional executive committee, and that she devoted a lot of her free time to union issues. Julia still couldn't understand why the young nursing assistants would want to join a union when relations with Westview's management seemed quite friendly and it cost so much to belong, or why Hattie thought the union was so important. While Julia and Hattie talked frequently, and Julia thought that Hattie liked her, Julia never discussed the union with her.

• • •

Hattie punched out for lunch at 1:05 p.m. and went straight to the staff room, where employees could eat. It contained several tables and chairs, a microwave, and a refrigerator, but lacked comfortable furniture.

Hattie wanted to straighten out the union bulletin board that hung there. She frequently posted articles about labor disputes and wanted to display a newspaper article about the recent National Labor Relations

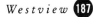

Board (NLRB) decision in favor of union members against the Ortho Nursing Home.

According to the NLRB ruling, Ortho had not provided the required financial information to the union or bargained in good faith. While the NLRB was ordering Ortho to do a number of things, the article also said Ortho would appeal. Hattie knew it would be at least a year before this would be resolved and "it was clearly too early to celebrate."

Hattie first learned about Ortho's situation from a woman who worked there. To show her support, Hattie frequently wore a button that said "Tough Times Don't Last, Tough People Do—1233."

Hattie punched back in at 1:55 p.m. First, she delivered the "health shakes" to those who needed vitamin supplements. She also delivered a health shake to Miss Szabo, who wasn't on the list but always wanted one, and made sure Miss Szabo could find her copy of *Szabadsag*, the Hungarian-language newspaper. Hattie caters to her because she knows that no one in her family comes to see Ms. Szabo and Hattie is "her company." Hattie also had to chase after Mrs. Juranyi to make sure she used her walker. Mrs. Juranyi doesn't like to use it, but Hattie was firm (again) about the doctor's orders. Hattie didn't want her to fall.

Hattie went to the nurse's station to get a list of questions to ask various residents. Some had to have blood pressure or temperature taken and all needed to be asked if they had had bowel movements and whether those had been small, medium, or large. Ms. Szabo said she hadn't had a bowel movement and was worried about that. Mr. Kundtz had wet his bed and muttered that Hattie should get her "fat ass in here now and clean the bed." He needed help washing, and his sheets had to be changed.

On her way back to the nurse's station, Hattie passed Julia Zrencsik, the young administrator, in the hall. Julia was talking with a resident and a nursing aide about some administrative procedure. Hattie often saw Julia take "a minute out to talk with folks." She liked Julia, even if her last name was totally unpronounceable, and had mentioned to others that "even if the administrators just walk around carrying papers, we are all doing the same work—caring for the residents."

Hattie met at 3:10 with the nursing assistant who just came on duty and would take her place. Hattie brought her up-to-date on the residents before she punched out at 3:30 p.m. She checked with Connie once more to make sure she knew where the meeting would be held and that she would go with one of the dietary aides who was also on the negotiating team.

. . .

Susan Haines and Harold Haines, a married couple, have owned and operated the Westview Nursing Home for 13 years. They are white and in their 50s, as are the attorney and the accountant who are their silent co-owners. When Harold, Susan, and their partners bought the home, the union was already in place.

Harold takes care of business arrangements for the home and Susan runs the day-to-day operation. Both are college graduates, but only she is a licensed nursing home administrator. He always wanted to get the license but never felt he had time to undertake the traineeship in another institution.

When Susan and Harold took over the home, management's relations with the union were very bad. Every contract negotiation had been painful. The employees felt little commitment to the home, employee turnover was high, and the previous owner had spent little time in the facility. Surveys called attention to numerous deficiencies and there was a large number of part-time employees. The professional staff was very unhappy with the way the owner gave orders, and publicly berated the entire staff.

The nursing home is much different now. It still has 154 beds, but the occupancy rate has increased to about 93 percent. The residents are 97 percent white and the payment structure is 18 percent private, 10 percent Medicare, and the rest Medicaid. The 160 employees are 91 percent female and 82 percent African American. Fifty percent of the employees are union members. The for-profit home recently won an award for excellence from a professional organization. The owners are interested in keeping a standard of excellence, and that includes continuing to have a good working relationship with their union.

Harold always has been a very direct person who tended to be a bit more assertive than necessary. The couple agreed many years ago that Susan would deal with the staff, resolve personnel problems, and negotiate with the union. She enjoyed "hanging out" with the staff, regularly went shopping with one union delegate, and would show up for staff softball games.

The owners began preparing for the contract negotiation in October. They reviewed the home's financial situation, discussed prospects, and identified problems. The financial condition was sound, but they were concerned that almost all the residents were Hungarian-Americans from the surrounding neighborhood and that the neighborhood's population base had shifted. They knew most residents' relatives liked the home's location because they worked downtown and could visit the home during their lunch period or after work. The owners thought Westview needed to do some marketing to expand their patient base, and they had asked Julia to help them do that.

Among the demands the owners identified to be included in their first contract proposal were the following:

- The day off one gets for one's birthday must be used within a one-month period, rather than anytime during the year.
- The probationary period for employees should be 75 days instead of 45 days.
- No buttons or other symbols of union affiliation could be worn when employees are in uniform.
- The owners would be allowed to give merit pay (bonuses) when the situation warranted.

The owners expected no difficulty with the first two issues, but thought the last two might not be acceptable to the union.

Susan usually is at work by midmorning, but today she arrives in the early afternoon because she worked a good part of the third shift last night. She does this every so often to make sure she is available to all the employees, not just those who work during the day. Susan tries to get Harold to do this, without much success, but Julia is scheduled periodically to work second and third shifts.

• • •

Paula Brown, a 45-year-old African American woman, is the 1233 organizer in the city. Her employer is the largest union of health care workers in the country. Its 425,000 members include nurses, medical technicians, physicians and home service workers. Paula was a nursing assistant at a long-term care facility for 12 years before taking on the area's organizing effort. One of her responsibilities is to handle the union's contract negotiations at seven "shops" (nursing homes). She contacted Westview in October to notify them that the union was interested in negotiating a new contract. Westview is a union shop, all full-time staff in the covered areas are required to join the union.

Paula talked with Westview's lawyer and administrator to schedule an initial meeting and the four meetings they expected would follow. She also called a meeting of Westview's unionized employees at the union hall. The employees elected a negotiating committee and came up with a list of contract demands. Some demands were suggested by Paula, based on information from the national and state offices, and others were suggested by those attending the meeting.

The union's state office supplies Paula with a Medicaid reimbursement report for Westview based on information available from the state government. The state and national offices also provide additional research information that may help Paula in the negotiating process, and an organizer from the state office would come out to work with her at any point if she wanted assistance.

Periodically, Paula goes to union-sponsored training sessions and seminars. One recent speaker discussed the globalization of business and how this has allowed employers to explicitly or implicitly threaten to relocate offices and plants. An organizer from another union talked about what to do when businesses hired "labor consultants" (union busters). Another speaker stressed that union movements rise and fade and that unionization is growing again in a form tailored to the new organizational structures. One university professor took the view that worker participation is not a democratizing movement if it is undertaken in the absence of a union. Another session provided some demographic information about unions in the United States and reminded participants that two out of every five union members are women, about 25 percent of African American women workers are unionized, and women who belong to unions make 83 percent of men's earnings, while working women as a whole make only 72 percent.[1]

Paula relies a lot on the delegate system to get the union's work done. Delegates are elected by members of each unionized group. The delegates receive extensive training so they can run predisciplinary hearings, deal with grievances, and represent the union, if necessary, in labor-management discussions. Many of the members of the negotiating committee are delegates.

• • •

Hattie arrives just in time for the caucus. She had to make one quick stop at the bank after work. She needed to take care of her rent payment, and her son had just given her his share of the money. (Hattie has lived in her home for 12 years and would like to buy it, but does not have the money to do so. One of her sons has moved back into the house, with his wife and daughter, and they are helping with expenses. If they stay long enough, she hopes to save enough for the down payment.)

The union caucus is held in the negotiation room. During the 45-minute caucus, union members are reminded about how the process works and they discuss the kinds of things that can be said during this first meeting. Any questions a committee member might have are answered by the organizer or other committee members. Connie asks why they are meeting in the lawyer's office. One union delegate reminds Connie that the group agreed to this location at their initial meeting. When the caucus ends, the door is opened and management is invited to join the union's negotiation team.

Before the meeting begins, those attending eat the food that has been provided. (The cost of refreshments is shared by management and labor.) Connie notices that Susan does not have anything to drink or eat and asks Susan if she could get something for her. One union delegate takes Connie aside and quietly lets her know she shouldn't be doing that at this type of meeting.

There is a large rectangular table in the room. Union representatives occupy three sides of the table if their group is large, or sit opposite management if their group is small. The union negotiation team is led by Paula Brown. In addition, a union representative from the state office in Columbus and all members of the home's negotiating team will be at the table. Usually the union at Westview has six to nine members on the negotiating team. Westview's administrator, Susan, is on the other side of the table. She is accompanied by her assistant administrator, Julia, and the organization's lawyer.

The meeting may be opened by either side. This time it is management's lawyer who thanks them all for coming and asks each person to introduce her- or himself. He also distributes a sign-in sheet. After the introductions, Paula says the union group is prepared to review its proposals.

The list she distributes is divided into two sections: non-economic items and economic items. Each item refers to the appropriate section of the contract. This year's list contains about 20 items, including:

- Establishment of a health and safety committee with representation from management and labor
- A political action check-off option that can be deducted automatically from a worker's check
- No reassignment of duties between job classifications
- A two-year contract instead of the present three-year contract
- Union orientation for new hires
- Comfortable furniture, including a couch, in the staff room
- Flu shots provided by the employer at no cost to employees
- Free meals while at work
- The possibility of enrolling in the 401K plan offered to all nonunion employees over one year ago
- Health insurance enrollment after 90 days of employment instead of 120 days
- A substantial wage increase.

The union does not expect to obtain all of the items on the list, but is putting them on the table for discussion. During the first meeting the union will briefly explain each item and answer questions to clarify why an item was included. Management will respond briefly to the list at the next meeting, and then present its list or a revised contract.

The list the union presents is not very specific, particularly in regard to economic issues, but will get more detailed over the course of the meetings. After the general points are made by both sides in the first and second meetings, the next meetings will deal in detail with noneconomic issues, and the last meetings will focus on economic issues.

The rest of the initial meeting is spent confirming dates and times for the next contract meetings. It often is difficult to coordinate the schedules of all the parties and so this phase takes some time.

• • •

After the initial contract meeting ends, Susan talks briefly with Westview's lawyer and then with Julia. Susan suggests that Julia meet with her tomorrow afternoon because she would like to hear Julia's thoughts about the meeting. Susan asks Julia to provide assistance to the lawyer by shaping management's response to the union list and justifying the items on management's list. Julia, pleased that Susan has so much confidence in her, agrees to help. She promises to have a first draft for discussion at their meeting the next day.

When Julia leaves the building, she notices that Hattie is waiting at the bus stop. Julia tells Hattie she is going to her mother's house on the East Side and would be happy to give her a ride home. Hattie accepts. There is so much that Julia would like to discuss with her.

Note

1. Tiffany, C., and L. R. Johnson Lutjen. 1993. "Pay Equity: It's Still With Us." *Journal of Professional Nursing*, 9 (January–February): 50–55.

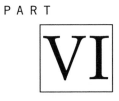

Program and Financial Development

Clark Retirement Community: Master Facility Plan Financing and Implementation

Donna D. VanIwaarden

BOB PERL gazed at the tiny structures in the model delivered by the architect earlier that day. After four years of strategic planning, feasibility studies, market research, consultations, negotiations, revisions, and countless committee meetings, the master plan was ready for implementation. It was an exciting plan that would literally turn the campus around. Over the next five years, a new entrance would be created, old facilities would be drastically renovated, and three-and-one-half acres of land, 38 townhomes, and a new nursing center would be added to the campus. All he needed now was $18 million!

History and Background

The Clark Retirement Community in Grand Rapids, Michigan, began operation in 1906 when Mr. and Mrs. M. J. Clark donated their farm to the Methodist Church to be used as a retirement home for ministers and deacons. Over the years the mission of the home broadened to include the laity, and it presently provides a continuum of services for the elderly ranging from skilled nursing care to independent apartment living for 358 residents. Clark has retained its church

---

The actual experiences of Clark Retirement Community in financing major capital improvement are described in this case.

affiliation, and its Board of Trustees and the majority of residents are United Methodists.

Clark consists of several well-maintained red brick buildings on a beautifully landscaped 12.5-acre site in a mature neighborhood. The focal point, a large, three-and-one-half story central building, is licensed for 229 "home for the aged" beds and 39 skilled nursing care beds. It is connected by a tunnel to a two-and-one-half story nursing center providing skilled care for an additional 72 residents. There are also nine independent living units located on the property—a fourplex, two duplexes and a cottage. Visitors to the Clark facilities are impressed by the vitality of the atmosphere, the availability of activities and amenities, and the warm, respectful treatment of residents.

Clark is a continuing care retirement community that is regulated by the Corporations and Securities Bureau of the Michigan Department of Commerce. It is a nonprofit corporation with an appraised insurable value of approximately $16 million. At every level of care in the continuum, Clark maintains high occupancy. Net operating revenue was $5,025,000 for the last fiscal year, and nonoperating revenue (income from contributions and interest on investments) was nearly $800,000. Revenues over expenses amounted to nearly $400,000. Clark has no long-term debt.

In addition to a monthly service charge based on level of care or accommodation, an entrance fee is required upon admission. Entrance fees are refunded on a prorated basis if an individual leaves the facility in less than five-and-one-half years. Residents may transfer to a higher level of care if their health status deteriorates. Once admitted to Clark, residents are not discharged because of inability to pay the monthly rate. Over 40 percent of the residents in the skilled nursing facility are on Medicaid. Since Medicaid reimbursement does not cover the full cost of care, Clark subsidizes this shortfall with its "benevolent care" fund. Last year that amount was nearly $400,000, which was paid from charitable contributions and interest earned on investments of reserve accounts.

Chief executive officer Bob Perl has been with Clark for six years. From the beginning of his tenure, the board has been talking about expansion. Bob agreed that it was needed, but wanted to proceed cautiously. He believed that it was imperative to gain the trust of residents, employees, and board members before undertaking a major expansion program. He also wanted to be sure that the institution was strong financially and organizationally. Over the past two years, he had succeeded on both accounts. His commitment to Clark's values and philosophy permeated the organization as he guided it through the long planning process culminating in the beautiful architectural model sitting in his office.

Planning for Expansion

Four years ago, a comprehensive strategic planning process resulted in a commitment to expand Clark Retirement Community's services and to renovate the campus. Because the campus was landlocked, initial plans called for expansion to a second location. The new site was found about five miles from the current campus. It appeared to be an ideal location for the development of an independent living complex, but required rezoning before plans could proceed. The property was adjacent to a small Christian liberal arts college. It seemed to offer exciting potential for "creative retirement" with intergenerational activities and opportunities for intellectual and artistic stimulation. After months of unsuccessful negotiations with the city planning board, Clark sadly dropped its option to purchase the land.

Disappointment faded when a longtime friend and benefactor stepped forward and donated a beautiful suburban property for the new campus. Once again, however, rezoning was required for the development of a multiunit retirement complex. When rezoning efforts failed for the second time, Clark's leadership began to reconsider the feasibility of developing the current campus.

Bob Perl called on a national specialist in retirement communities and services for the elderly from the United Methodist Church. For nearly five months the consultant led the board and staff through the process of evaluating the needs of the present campus. The following seven conclusions were reached:

1. Although the aging campus was well-maintained, individual accommodations at every service level were too small.
2. Having skilled nursing care in two buildings connected by a tunnel was inefficient and ineffective.
3. More assisted living units were needed to meet increased demand.
4. Adding more independent living units would invigorate and revitalize the campus. These units could be built at the present location, but would be extremely price- and market-sensitive.
5. Clark Retirement Community was probably the best-kept secret in town. It was known by the Methodist constituency, but not by the local community.
6. Clark needed to build new facilities and renovate all current space, and the project should be done in phases over a period of years.
7. The development of a second campus in a suburban location should remain in the long-range plan.

Agreement on the findings brought renewed commitment to developing the Clark campus. A flurry of planning activity followed.

Development of the Master Plan

The decision to proceed with a major capital investment in the Clark campus meant organizing and activating board and staff to gather information. Many critical decisions regarding the configuration of new facilities and the remodeling of old ones would have to be made. Expansion plans needed to be designed to meet market demands at competitive rates. Overinvestment or underinvestment could jeopardize the long-term viability of the organization.

New building and finance committees were activated and inquiries were made regarding the possibility of purchasing land surrounding the campus. A three-and-one-half acre tract adjoining Clark's property was available, and negotiations were initiated to acquire it. Members of the board and staff toured state-of-the-art retirement communities in a nearby state. One of those communities proved to be particularly intriguing, since its creative design fully utilized a comparatively small site.

When the CEO returned from that visit, he checked the references of the architect who designed the Ohio project. Good reports confirmed Bob's own intuitive judgment. He was convinced that Clark should bring the Ohio architect to Grand Rapids to explore options for their own small campus. When Bob met with the board and made his recommendation, they were reluctant at first. There were fine architects in the local area. Why go to the additional expense of bringing in someone from out of state? Ultimately, they put their trust in Bob's judgment and approved his recommendation. It turned out to be one of their best decisions.

Bob contacted the architect and described Clark's small campus and big dreams. After several preparatory telephone and written communications, the architect visited Clark Retirement Community. In only a few hours, he had sketched a dramatic new vision for campus development. With acquisition of the three-and-one-half acre parcel, the campus could literally be turned around to "face the twenty-first century!" The site plan called for independent living townhomes to be built near the new entrance along a tree-lined winding road. This road would lead to the existing structures with the addition of a new three-story nursing center in the heart of the campus, a solution no one had thought of before.

A demographic study of the neighborhood confirmed that to have the new entrance on Franklin Street would be desirable. The area to the west and north of the campus was aging and deteriorating. Franklin Street was an attractive, wide boulevard lined with large, well-maintained homes and other buildings. In addition to being aesthetically more appealing, the four lane boulevard could handle traffic better than the neighborhood street currently used to serve Clark.

Working directly with staff and listening to their programming requirements, the architect developed comprehensive space plans. Within four months he had changed the location of every service except dietary and purchasing. His creative scheme embodied the Clark dream and brought renewed vitality and excitement to the project.

With a creative new site plan in place, the next step was to determine how many independent living units should be built. An extensive market research project was initiated. Survey respondents and focus group participants were enthusiastic in their support of Clark's proposed development. They believed it offered what they wanted—a lifestyle of comfort, security, and affordability. Based on the research, the units could be designed to satisfy customer preferences for floor plans, amenities, and price ranges.

The accelerated pace of activities continued with the hiring of a local architectural firm experienced in projects for the elderly. With the cooperative efforts of the architect, board, staff, and committees, the master plan began to emerge. After a seemingly endless number of revisions, the final plan was unveiled. It consisted of a five-year project to be implemented in four phases at a cost of $18 million.

The first phase to be constructed would be the independent living units—38 single-story brick townhomes to be called Clark Commons. Based on data gathered in the focus groups and other competitor analyses, three basic floor plans were developed. All homes included attached garages, rear patios, major appliances, and 24-hour emergency call systems. The units would range in price from $75,000 to $89,000. The total cost of Phase I would be $3.5 million.

Phase II would be the construction of a new 111-bed nursing center close to everyone, at the center of the campus. It would contain 75 private rooms and 18 semi-private rooms designed as "living clusters," rather than the typical series of rooms off of a main hallway. Each cluster would be comprised of eight to ten rooms grouped around a living/dining/relaxation area. A "main street" would occupy the first floor, providing amenities for the entire community. The cost of this phase was set at $9 million.

Renovation and updating of the older facilities comprised Phase 3, to take place in the fourth year of the project. The current two-and-one-half story nursing center would be converted into 44 one-bedroom apartments for retirement residents, at a cost of $3.5 million.

The final phase would be the renovation of the large central building, to become the future Assisted Living Center. This involved remodeling and updating all of the current spaces, thereby increasing the number of accommodations from 48 to 100. Cost for this phase would be $2 million.

Financing the Project

While the architect developed preliminary sketches and cost estimates, the finance committee explored financing options. Four sources of capital financing were identified as follows:

1. *Charitable contributions.* Because of the nonprofit status of the organization, its good reputation, and its association with the Methodist Church, a major fundraising effort was a distinct possibility. There had been no major capital campaigns or fundraising efforts in recent years. The local congregations of the United Methodist Church and the families and friends of past residents of Clark were identified as potential donors.

2. *Pre-sale of the independent living units.* Competitor analysis revealed that other senior living projects in the metropolitan area had successfully used this type of financing. Selling the new townhomes prior to construction would raise most of the capital needed to finance Phase I.

3. *Use of reserves.* Clark maintained fairly substantial reserves for funding benevolent care and capital replacement. Restructuring these reserves could release funds for construction without jeopardizing benevolent care.

4. *Long-term debt (borrowing).* There were three possibilities for long-term financing: conventional mortgage, Federal Housing Administration (FHA)-insured mortgage, and tax-exempt revenue bonds. This was clearly the most costly form of financing. However, Clark was in a good position to consider debt financing, since it currently had no long-term debt.

With the assistance of the finance committee, the business and finance director and the CEO began detailed exploration of the feasibility of the various options.

Capital Campaign

Fundraising can be an important source of capital for non-profit organizations. In 1992, private giving in the United States totaled over $124 billion. Over the years, Clark has been a beneficiary of this philanthropic spirit, regularly receiving about $350,000 a year from its supporters.

Charitable contributions represented the most inexpensive form of capital financing for Clark, but a successful capital campaign still requires diligent preplanning. A consultant was hired to determine the feasibility of a major capital campaign. The study involved confidential interviews with forty individuals selected from board members, church and civic leaders, business executives, and residents and friends of Clark. The consultant reported that Clark had a reputation for high-quality compassionate care, and that the master plan project was universally perceived as progressive and appropriate.

Critical prerequisites for a successful capital campaign were in place: (1) a good donor base, (2) an important cause, (3) a reputation for high-quality programs, and (4) effective board and campaign leadership. The consultant recommended a target objective of $2,250,000. Clark's development officer carefully evaluated the precampaign analysis and prepared a tentative 18-month campaign schedule and a preliminary budget.

In a well-designed, disciplined fundraising plan, efforts are made to secure large gifts early in the campaign. This gives momentum to the cause and encouragement to potential donors. The leadership of the Clark campaign identified prospects for large gifts. The first solicitation resulted in a $1 million gift from a longtime Clark supporter! With this generous contribution, the campaign was up and running with great enthusiasm. In fact, the leaders began to reconsider their original objective. Was it too low? Should they set their sights on a higher goal?

Pre-sale of Townhomes

In examining pre-sale financing of the townhomes, the finance committee reviewed similar projects in the metropolitan area. They found that most potential buyers owned their homes and would be willing and able to use their equity to purchase a townhome. In this form of creative financing, buyers "prepay" the purchase price of their townhome, which produces for the institution the cash required for construction.

The pre-sale financing plan required that 60 percent of the townhomes be sold before construction could begin. Buyers would each make a down payment of $1,000 to reserve their home, and the remainder of the mortgage note amount would be paid incrementally within 210 days after construction started. When construction was completed, the buyers would sign a residency agreement. Under the terms of this agreement, 70 percent of the purchase price would be refunded when residents left or transferred to other Clark facilities. If a buyer decided not to sign a residency agreement, Clark would repay the mortgage note within 12 months.

This pre-sale financing plan, known as the sale of noninterest bearing mortgage notes, required the filing of a prospectus with the state securities and exchange commission detailing the terms, obligations, and risks of all parties involved. The costs associated with raising the $3.5 million to build the Clark Commons townhomes, excluding marketing expenses, was estimated to be $35,000. This amount included legal fees and a financing fee to the bank for a trust mortgage. The trust mortgage would secure the repayment of the mortgage notes if required.

This plan would allow Clark to finance Phase I without incurring debt or depleting its internal reserves. The preliminary work was done, the marketing materials were prepared, and construction was set to begin in nine months. Could the required number of homes be sold in such a short time?

Use of Internal Reserves

Clark maintains reserves of over $4 million from retained earnings and endowments. Interest earned on reserves is used to fund benevolent care and capital expenditures. The corporation is also self-insured for workers' compensation claims up to $275,000, and maintains reserves for refundable entrance fees.

One function of a board is to determine the amount of money held in reserve. With board approval, money from reserves could be used to finance campus construction. The loss of earned interest would be offset somewhat by the reduced cost of borrowing additional capital. At current interest rates, the differential would be about 2 percent. How much money from reserves could be used for construction without jeopardizing benevolent care and other obligations?

Tax-Exempt Bond Financing

As the committee investigated long-term financing options they quickly learned that tax-exempt bond financing would be less expensive than either conventional or FHA loans. Bonds are similar to loans in that a borrower agrees to make principal and interest payments on specific dates to the holder of the bond. Because interest earned on these bonds is exempt from federal income taxation, their coupon (interest) rate is about 2 percent lower than that of other sources of capital.

The process of bond financing involves many different entities. A public issuing authority is required for tax-exempt bonds, in addition to underwriters, bankers, attorneys, and bond buyers. In order to obtain a lower interest rate on the bonds, Clark could ask for a "letter of credit" from its bank, known as a credit enhancement. For a 1 percent fee, the bank would assume the risk of default, giving the bond a rating of AA. This excellent rating would enhance the attractiveness of the bonds to potential buyers, making it easier to sell them. In exchange for a letter of credit, Clark would pledge its assets to the bank as security for the bond indebtedness.

Fortunately for Clark, interest rates were at the lowest they had been in 17 years. The bank agreed to provide the letter of credit, but there were several other options to be considered. Both variable and fixed rate financing were available. With variable rate financing, the initial interest rate would be lower, but it could increase substantially over the life of the bonds. A fixed rate would mean predictable principal and interest payments, and no unexpected hikes in resident rates to cover added interest expense.

How much should the bond issue be, and how should it be structured?

Financial Projections

Before going into debt, an organization must determine whether income will be sufficient to cover the added principal and interest payments. This requires forecasts of income and expenses based on realistic assumptions about census and staffing levels, inflation, acceptable rate increases, donations, and investment income. The CEO's overriding concern was the effect of the debt on the rate structure. The higher the cost of capital, the higher the rates for services would have to be set. Organizational viability required that rates remain competitive at every service level and that operating revenues be sufficient to repay the indebtedness.

Based on careful consideration of potential funding from the capital campaign, restructuring of reserves, and the pre-sale of the independent living units, a bond issue of $10,500,000 seemed to be realistic and appropriate. Proposals were solicited from four investment banking firms and the director of business and finance began a detailed analysis of the financial information.

First, he set up a database using a computerized spreadsheet so it would be possible to easily examine a number of alternatives. As shown in Table 17.1, he entered expected census at each care level, the projected number of full-time equivalents (employees) required to provide services, and current resident rates.

Using historical data and economic predictions for the local region, assumptions were made about annual inflation (6 percent for salaries and wages, 5.5 percent for fringe benefits, 5 percent for purchased services, 6.2 percent for supplies) and nonoperating revenue (10 percent increase in donations, 1.5 percent increase in investment income).

Acceptable annual rate increases were also determined (3.5 percent for independent living and retirement residents, 10 percent for assisted

Table 17.1 Expected Census, Projected FTEs, and Current Rates

	Year 1	Year 2	Year 3	Year 4	Year 5
Average Census					
Independent living	15	48	48	48	48
Resident	169	153	138	138	138
ALC	44	58	71	71	71
Nursing	109	109	109	109	109
Monthly Rate					
Independent living	$ 751	$ 429	$ 444	$ 460	$ 476
Resident	$ 780	$ 807	$ 835	$ 864	$ 894
ALC	$1,200	$1,320	$1,452	$1,597	$1,756
Nursing	$2,354	$2,531	$2,721	$2,925	$3,144
Total FTE employees	182	188	189	192	192

Table 17.2 Pro Forma Operating Revenues and Expenses

	Year 1	Year 2	Year 3	Year 4	Year 5
Operating Revenues					
Resident services	$5,429,652	$5,958,024	$6,434,676	$6,882,288	$7,363,956
Entrance fees	$ 286,911	$ 340,932	$ 340,932	$ 340,932	$ 340,932
Other operating	$ 57,430	$ 59,440	$ 61,520	$ 63,674	$ 65,902
Total operating revenues	$5,773,993	$6,358,396	$6,837,128	$7,286,894	$7,770,790
Operating Expenses					
Salaries and wages	$3,445,324	$3,772,438	$4,020,054	$4,328,896	$4,588,630
Fringe benefits	$ 639,470	$ 696,884	$ 739,124	$ 792,154	$ 835,722
Purchased services	$ 139,714	$ 146,700	$ 154,035	$ 161,737	$ 169,824
Supplies and other	$1,420,626	$1,508,705	$1,602,245	$1,701,584	$1,807,082
Total operating expenses	$5,645,134	$6,124,727	$6,515,458	$6,984,371	$7,401,258

living, and 7.5 percent for skilled nursing). The rate for the independent living units would change to $429 per month in the second year of the project. This was calculated as a weighted average based on the rental rates of the old units plus the monthly fees for the new townhomes. With these data, it was possible to prepare pro forma (projected) financial statements for the five years of the project, as shown in Table 17.2.

According to the terms of the bond issue, payback of principal and interest would begin in the fourth year of the project. In that year, and every year thereafter for the next 20 years, the payment would be approximately $1 million. From the projected financial statements it was clear that revenues would be insufficient to meet the principal and interest payment. To make the debt payment, resident service rates would have to be increased. A competitive analysis of area resident rates was conducted to determine the feasibility of a rate increase for Clark.

Rates for all four levels of care were collected from 17 nursing homes and retirement communities. The data revealed that monthly fees for independent living were about the same for all providers. However, Clark was significantly lower in the rates for all other levels of care. Clark was particularly interested in the data from two nearby retirement communities which were the most comparable to it in services, amenities, and market niche. The comparative data are provided in Table 17.3. Clearly, Clark could raise rates to cover the $1 million debt payment and still be competitive. The question left was—What should the flat rate increase be for each level of care?

Current Status

Bob Perl gazed out the window and surveyed the tulips forming a colorful display in the front (but soon to be back) courtyard, and reflected on the work that had already been accomplished. How many meetings had he attended, he wondered. Too many to count, he supposed, but using committees had been advantageous to the process. Committees were inherently part of the Methodist culture and they worked well to build consensus and participation. Committee members had been chosen on the basis of their leadership effectiveness, their credibility with the organization, and their expertise in specific areas useful to the project. They had worked well, and Bob had learned to keep the committees focused, giving his staff responsibility for the details. Good staff support was essential, and he had a good staff.

Table 17.3   Rates

	Retirement (per month)	Assisted Living (per month)	Nursing (per day)
Manor X	$910	$1,725	$106
Village Y	$900–$1,450	$1,600	$ 95 (semi-private) $130 (private)
Clark	$780	$1,200	$ 76 (semi-private) $ 86 (private)

Throughout the long planning process, Bob had maintained an excellent working relationship with his board and staff. He kept them well-informed and updated. Board members received minutes from all committee meetings and copies of consultant reports. Staff conferred directly with the consultants, providing their own specific expertise relating to programming and services. Bob attended resident council meetings to answer questions and reassure residents about the plans for Clark. Once construction got underway, he planned to write a weekly newsletter to keep residents and employees informed on the progress of construction and renovation.

From all of the planning he had done so far, Bob had learned that working with consultants could be difficult. Some of them seemed to have a tendency to tell their clients what they wanted to hear; it was important to keep pushing for results. Consultants also were expensive, so they had to be used effectively. Doing that required three things: (1) checking backgrounds and references to get good consultants, (2) a clear idea of what needed to be accomplished, and (3) having consultants work directly with members of the staff. Bob thought of the creative architect from Ohio who had designed the site and space plans. His work had turned out to be one of the best overall values in consulting services.

Bob perused the reports on his desk, wondering where all this was going to take him. Tonight he would make his final recommendation to the board on the $18 million financing package. He had carefully studied the data, but the financial projections were based on assumptions. Were those assumptions accurate? Had he missed anything in the analysis? How would the board react to his recommendations?

ConstantCaring: Managed Medical Care in the Nursing Home

Margaret Hastings

Introduction

WITH BURGEONING Medicare costs, Congress passed the Tax Equity and Fiscal Responsibility Act in 1982 (TEFRA) that included important amendments to Medicare. These amendments permitted risk contracting with licensed HMOs to provide, under a capitated contract, all services covered under Medicare Parts A and B for enrolled beneficiaries. The goal was to improve continuity of care, preventive services, case management, and quality of care while controlling costs. In recent years, five percent of Medicare beneficiaries participated in one of these TEFRA capitated managed care programs.

Continuing concern about the quality of medical care in long-term care facilities was addressed with the passage of the Omnibus Budget Reconciliation Act of 1987 (OBRA '87). This comprehensive nursing home reform mandated uniform assessment of residents and care planning, upgrading of staff requirements and training, new responsibilities for physicians in caring for residents, and for medical directors to oversee resident care.

Several studies and assessments have identified the problems of adequately trained and experienced medical personnel in caring for the medical needs of an increasingly disabled nursing home population. Specialized programs have been developed to respond to this need. From

This case is based on actual experiences with implementation of managed care models in nursing homes. Names, events, and locations have been altered for purposes of teaching and confidentiality.

1982 to 1987 the W. K. Kellogg Foundation supported a demonstration program involving some 150 nursing homes in 12 western states in an effort to improve the quality of nursing home services through the use of geriatric nurse practitioners (GNPs). The model involved the selection of a well-respected staff nurse who would complete an academic program leading to certification as a GNP and complete a practicum at the employing nursing facility. These nurses worked with all residents, applying their advanced practice and gerontological nursing skills, with the support of attending physicians. The program was highly successful and demonstrated the advantages of employing GNPs in these settings (Grace et al. 1988).

These two major federal policy initiatives (TEFRA '82 and OBRA '87), along with studies and demonstrations like those supported by the W. K. Kellogg Foundation, form the backdrop for this case. The setting involves a managed care program designed to improve the quality of medical services for nursing home residents while, at the same time, limiting copayment liabilities for residents and their families.

The ConstantCaring Model

A for-profit health care corporation offering several HMO products developed an innovative use of the TEFRA Medicare risk contract. A young executive in the firm, who was also a nurse practitioner, developed a new managed care product designed to provide medical services in nursing homes. The product met OBRA '87 standards for medical care while eliminating inappropriate hospitalizations and emergency room episodes. The services emphasize case management, primary care and preventive services, communication and work with families, and the use of advance directives.

The program, called ConstantCaring (CC), restructures medical care delivery and financing for enrolled nursing home residents. The program uses physician and geriatric nurse practitioner teams to provide medical care. Capitated risk-based financing of all Medicare-covered services provides more flexible use of funds paid to the provider organization under the TEFRA risk contract. The Medicare payment level to the provider is determined based on the adjusted average per capita cost (AAPCC) of providing Medicare services in the area. The payment rate also varies based on additional factors, such as the individual's age, gender, and institutional status.

Geriatric nurse practitioners (GNPs) in the CC program act as case managers for medical services to enrolled nursing home residents. They concentrate on prevention, early intervention, and quality of life, thus reducing unnecessary care. After performing an assessment on new members of the CC program, the GNP develops a care plan, with physician involvement and family consultation. GNPs conduct all routine visits, at least monthly, during and after which they evaluate progress, conduct examinations, and coordinate with facility staff. They must preauthorize hospitalizations and appointments with specialists, and are available on a 24-hour basis. They also have constant access to consultation and supervision by their geriatrician partner. GNPs can either be under contract or salaried, depending on their level of involvement in the program.

CC pays primary care physicians substantially above Medicare reimbursement rates as an incentive to participate in the program. Using a modified fee-for-service schedule, they are reimbursed for unlimited primary care and urgent care visits in the nursing home, case management, and family and consultant conferences. However, physician office visits usually are not reimbursed. Specialty and hospital care is provided by the appropriate quality providers under contract with CC. Finally, any Medicare recipient who is a long-stay nursing home resident may join the program. No one is turned down due to their medical condition or prior history.

The ConstantCaring program was founded in a large western metropolitan area in a state known for high nursing home care standards. This state pays one of the highest Medicaid rates in the country and has a strong and innovative survey process. Requirements for administrators also are among the highest in the nation. To help launch the program, an advisory committee of state officials, nursing home leaders, and medical practitioners was formed to advise on marketing and operational matters.

In its first four years of operation, the CC membership experienced lower hospital utilization rates, shorter lengths of stay (average 4.5 days per admission), and more skilled nursing facility use than traditional Medicare fee-for-service participants. The program was found to improve access to and quality of medical care, while enhancing family and physician satisfaction. It was also viewed as a major force for quality medical care in nursing homes throughout the state. ConstantCaring demonstrated that it could provide access to appropriate medical care while controlling costs. With more than 800 enrollees, the plan was also profitable.

Based on this success, the corporation decided to replicate the model in a new site, called ConstantCaring2 (CC2). A major east coast city was selected because of its large number of nursing homes. Nursing home quality had been a statewide problem, especially in homes with a large percentage of Medicaid residents. Low Medicaid reimbursement rates and slow payment cycles made managing these Medicaid homes difficult.

ConstantCaring executives expected the new location to provide a great opportunity for the program. The metropolitan area had several medical schools with extensive interest in gerontology and clinical research on conditions of the elderly. Three nursing home associations were very active in the state legislative process. Physicians also had considerable political power. Of special note was the fact that the state had been slow to recognize physician assistants and geriatric nurse practitioners. Similarly, managed care was slow to penetrate the marketplace. ConstantCaring strategists felt there would be ample opportunity for their product, since it could enhance care with no additional cost to the state.

ConstantCaring2 Start-Up

Given the substantial opportunity and the apparent open market, Jenny Swanson, RN, NP, MPH, ConstantCaring's chief executive officer, secured space for ConstantCaring2 in a building where another division of the company was located, about 25 miles from the city's center. She quickly hired an operating room head nurse, Leeanne Lipinski, as project executive. Leeanne was a good friend of some of the nurses in the parent corporation and was known as a "no nonsense manager" with a "get the job done" style. She had little knowledge of long-term care or primary care services, and she was not a nurse practitioner.

While the office was being prepared for occupancy and initial contacts were made to contract with nurse practitioners and physicians, Jenny held several key meetings. At the state capitol she spoke with Dr. Whistle, who oversaw the nursing home survey process for the state department of health. Jenny described ConstantCaring2 and its goal of offering nursing home residents better access to quality medical care. She reviewed the membership process, case management procedures, and the operation of physician and nurse practitioner teams.

Dr. Whistle was pleased with the program, talking at length about how state surveyors reported frustration at facilities because nurses often could not reach a resident's physician. He thought the GNP primary care visits would prevent some of these crises and was pleased that CC2 contract physicians were geriatricians, always available to the GNP in coordinating the case.

Dr. Whistle also liked the idea that nursing home staff would not just send the resident to the hospital when a problem occurred on the understaffed night shift. Instead, the nursing home would contact the ConstantCaring2 GNP and physician team to assess the situation and find alternatives. He thought, however, that some hospitals, privately, might be against the Constant Caring program because they depended on hospitalizations from the nursing homes to address declining occupancy rates.

Dr. Whistle cautioned Jenny about the need for adhering to the state's more than 3,000 regulations for nursing homes; she should know that the days of nursing homes "getting by" were over. With five lawyers on his staff, nursing homes were in court almost every day relating to issues of regulatory compliance. He also thought she should know that the medical society was one of the most powerful groups in the state. They had substantial influence on the use of nurse practitioners and physician assistants. In fact, the state nurse practice act had only recently recognized advanced practice nursing, and the scope of practice for the nurse practitioner had not yet been identified. Based on the ConstantCaring model Jenny presented, Dr. Whistle offered to write a letter stating that the state health department had determined that the CC2 program met legal standards as long as nurse practitioners worked under physician supervision and did not prescribe medications. Copies of the letter could be made available to nursing homes with ConstantCaring2 members.

A few weeks after her visit to the Capitol, lawyers from the state medical society were reported to be advising their members against involvement with a program such as ConstantCaring because working as a team with nurse practitioners could increase their liability and, perhaps, their malpractice insurance premiums. Jenny was surprised by this reaction. The program had only begun discussions with a few geriatricians about contracting with ConstantCaring2 and the original program site had not generated this kind of professional opposition. Jenny set up an appointment the very next week to meet with medical society representatives to discuss the CC program and how it worked.

The New Executive Arrives

Once Leeanne moved to the area, she quickly set up the ConstantCaring2 office. She was very effective in organizing and completing the paperwork and developing office procedures. Another corporate subsidiary in the same market area, a licensed HMO called Healthwise, served as the fiscal intermediary for ConstantCaring2's billing and claims processing to meet Medicare risk-contracting requirements. Healthwise had 32,000 Medicare clients and was anxious for further expansion of its older adult membership.

Once the office was established, Leeanne began calling on nursing home administrators and medical directors to introduce herself and ConstantCaring2. After several meetings, she realized that her marketing message was being misunderstood. Administrators and physicians often became confused during her presentation, thinking that Leeanne was promoting some kind of long-term care insurance. She would then back up and clarify that the product included all Medicare-covered medical services, in or out of the facility, not long-term care room and board payments.

Obtaining ConstantCaring2 memberships became the top priority. Unfortunately, Leeanne found this to be difficult and was very frustrated with the slow progress of her marketing efforts. As a result, she increasingly focused her work on office operations, smooth claims processing, and the arduous paperwork entailed in enrolling new members. At the end of six months, five GNPs were under part-time contract to service thirty clients in fifteen nursing homes and seven physicians were working with the GNPs to form the primary care service teams.

Dr. Fairchild, a staff member of a leading academic medical center, also signed a contract to be CC2's part-time medical director. He was a young doctor with a primary care practice with little time to focus on ConstantCaring2 patients, but lent the good name of his medical center. He took on about eight CC2 clients in three nursing homes. Leeanne got complaints that he didn't follow up fast enough after residents entered the program, which she worried might cause noncompliance with physician visit regulations. Facility administrators were especially concerned about this issue.

Recognizing a Marketing Problem

Slow membership growth prompted Jenny to send an accomplished social worker, who also had marketing experience, to work on closing sales with nursing home residents and their families. New "leads" were generated through a variety of mechanisms including a telemarketing initiative run by Healthwise.

The new ConstantCaring2 marketing representative, Rachel Larson, was a perceptive woman who worked well with families. She had a knack for introducing the program to nursing home administrators and staff. However, many still reacted with suspicion when they heard about physician and GNP teams working with residents in their facilities. Rachel quickly discovered that she had to work twice as hard to cover for Leeanne's earlier brusk and impatient manner in her "get acquainted" calls.

Rachel's knowledge, good sense, and diplomacy enabled CC2 membership to grow despite these problems. Fortunately, Rachel thought, CC2 marketing supervision had been given to Judy Carlson, a telemarketing specialist who had recently moved to the East from corporate headquarters to take over the marketing of Healthwise. They became close friends and spent after-work hours together.

Leeanne's shortcomings in managing the new site of ConstantCaring were becoming more apparent. She was especially tired of nurse practitioners coming to her with questions about how they should handle difficult cases. Fortunately for Leeanne, a job more suited to her skills and interests became available at corporate headquarters.

Year Two: A New Director

Jenny was anxious not to lose valuable time in developing the new site. She appointed Naomi Kupperschmidt to succeed Leeanne as executive director. Although Naomi had little management or marketing experience, she was known at the corporate office as an excellent GNP who had superb clinical skills, got along well with nursing home personnel and physicians, and knew her way around the clinical service system in the area. Jenny felt Naomi would be excellent in controlling hospital utilization, a substantial problem during the first year of operation. Reducing hospital days is a key factor in building the new site toward financial viability.

Naomi's first action was to form an advisory committee similar to the one which had so successfully guided the original site. The committee included administrators, nurses, physicians, academicians, and representatives from the state government and area agencies on aging. At the first meeting Jenny flew in from corporate headquarters and laid out the product, its rationale, and described the success of the original program.

Naomi also quickly contracted with several geriatric physicians to handle the growing enrollment of about eight new cases per month. She was able to entice additional experienced and capable GNPs to work part-time, which cut down on travel times to CC2 members, who were now spread among 35 homes in three counties.

Naomi was anxious to see membership grow since her compensation and promotion opportunity were linked to program size. Increasingly, she thought that CC2 marketing should be under her control, not in another corporate division. When Rachel Larson, the CC2 marketing representative who worked under the direction of Judy Carlson, took another job out of the state, Naomi saw this as an opportunity to alter reporting relationships. But, Jenny, as CC chief executive, was reluctant to make a change because of complicated corporate senior executive interrelationships involving the leadership at Healthwise.

At this same time, Naomi became very concerned about the growing numbers of Healthwise managed care patients who were being transferred into CC2 when they had been in nursing homes for some time.

Typically they were very frail, had multiple needs, and were at extremely costly stages in their care. The patients often died within a few months after transfer. It was expensive, time consuming, and demoralizing to physicians and GNPs to bring these elders into CC2's program and transfer their Medicare rights, only to have them expire. These transfers, although increasing the membership numbers, were having a negative effect on the ConstantCaring2 balance sheet. As CC2's executive, Naomi personally felt the brunt of this dumping with the increased burden of orienting her staff to these new, often short-lived cases, working with residents' families, and interfacing with nursing home staffs with residents who frequently were in crisis.

Marketing: Can the Pieces Be Put Together?

In replacing the CC2 marketing person, Rachel Larson, Naomi argued again with CC corporate leadership for full control of ConstantCaring2's marketing program. Despite CC2 corporate concerns over reducing the Healthwise transfers and the need for specific new and different CC2 marketing initiatives, Naomi's bid was unsuccessful. Judy Carlson instead replaced Rachel with two new marketing representatives to cover the large metropolitan geographic area: Chloe had some marketing experience in real estate and Sarah, a nursing home social worker, was familiar with the CC2 product. Their training at corporate headquarters and orientation to CC took nearly three months. Although the program had grown to just over 100 members, only five new members signed up during that period.

As Chloe and Sarah began their full marketing efforts, confusion about who was their boss became apparent, especially because Judy Carlson knew relatively little about the nursing home market. In contrast, Naomi had in-depth knowledge of nursing homes, their leadership and idiosyncrasies, information critical in developing strategy and making successful calls. After a few months, Jenny made the decision to work with Healthwise senior executives to move the marketing responsibility to ConstantCaring2. She assigned supervision jointly to Naomi at CC2 and Linda Nelson at corporate headquarters, who had successfully marketed the original program.

Naomi assumed substantial responsibility for supervising the two marketing positions, while Linda often gave conflicting instructions, usually by phone, related to her marketing experiences at the original CC site. She wanted to impress Jenny with how effective she could be in applying her knowledge and skills to other CC sites. Linda had pushed hard at corporate headquarters for this new responsibility because she had heard that CC might expand to several different sites across the nation in the following year. Understandably, she wanted the additional pay and prestige a national sales director title would bring.

Even with elaborate corporate training and double supervision, the marketing representatives had trouble enrolling new members. Coached by Linda, they followed "leads" provided by telemarketing at Healthwise and from special events at local nursing homes sponsored by CC2. They spent endless hours driving to nursing homes and setting up informational visits with nursing staff, social workers, and administrators. They worked with activity directors to set up special events on Sundays and holidays, when family members could attend parties with the residents.

In spite of their energy and hospitality, they found that nursing home personnel still misunderstood the product, mistrusted them, or said their physicians didn't want a managed care plan doctor in the facility. Even when families realized that the $37.87 monthly copayment was the extent of their Medicare liability, there was still reluctance to join the program, especially if nursing home personnel were not supportive of the CC2 program.

Meeting with the Physicians: Assessing Progress

About nine months into the second year, Jenny came to the east coast to speak at a convention. Since she was available, meetings were set up with CC2 contract physicians and the advisory committee members. A luncheon was held for physicians to discuss their experiences. Two non-CC2 physicians were also invited so they could learn more about the program and explore potential interest in signing contracts.

In discussing how physicians liked working with CC2, Dr. Aylward said he originally had difficulty getting used to a new way of practicing, but now he enjoyed working with Anna White, his GNP partner, and felt that she was highly skilled. He liked the model with routine visits conducted by Anna. She relayed essential information to him and offered practical advice to the nursing home staff about improving patient care.

Jenny shared her concerns about handling resident emergencies and described the successful experience at the original site. To solve a growing CC2 emergency transportation problem, she felt they should contract directly with an ambulance company that would take the patient where CC2 wanted them to go. Currently, when an ambulance takes a CC2 resident from the nursing home to a hospital emergency room the patient could end up at any one of several local hospitals. If the CC2 physician on the case didn't practice there, it posed significant problems of time and expense to make a transfer or find another physician to see the patient temporarily. Physicians at the luncheon pointed out that the state Emergency Services Act required centralized control. Ambulance drivers had to take patients where they were told, which was determined by the patient's condition and the time estimated to reach the appropriate, critical care needed.

Dr. Yu, a carefully spoken and conscientious CC physician, felt that CC2 should only be offered in nursing homes meeting high standards and with superior nursing staffs. He identified two facilities where he didn't want any more CC2 members assigned to him because the staff seemed inept and did not follow his orders.

Dr. Green, a potential CC2 physician, brought his nurse, Ms. Bloom, with whom he practices in five nursing homes. He wondered if she would want to practice with the program. During the discussion, Jenny wrote a note to Naomi indicating that Ms. Bloom would not meet CC2 standards without added qualifications as a nurse practitioner, and she didn't want the model diluted by using RNs, which would run the risk of reducing the quality of service provided.

As the physician luncheon closed, Dr. Burton offered that he had learned from the CC model to concentrate much more on the patient's comfort and to order tests and medications more conservatively. He had also found the GNPs hired by CC2 to be of the highest caliber, and he had changed his mind about nurses being able to manage cases and work with families. Overall, the luncheon had been a success.

Community Advisory Committee Meeting

The second advisory committee meeting was called a few months later. It was a breakfast meeting at a noted club in the city. Committee members welcomed the cuisine and view. This time Jenny's comments focused on the problems she saw with CC2's development. Advisory committee members emphasized that the new CC site culture was different from that where the program had originally worked. Further development of CC2 could succeed only if marketing efforts were directed at physicians with nursing home practices, nursing home administrators and medical directors, and long-term care associations . . . they were the real customers. They emphasized that families wouldn't join a new program if they felt that their loved one might face repercussions in the nursing home because of resentment toward the CC2 personnel or the team approach.

Year Three: Time of Decision

During the following seven months, neither of the two new marketing representatives met their quota of ten new members per month. By late in the third year, the net enrollment had climbed to only 130 members. This was far short of the corporate plan's "break even" goal of 200 needed by year's end, only six weeks away.

A third advisory committee meeting was held two weeks later. Naomi welcomed the committee and outlined ongoing efforts to build an effective program. In addition to her position as CC2 executive director, staff working in the CC2 office now included one full-time and two half-time GNPs and an administrative coordinator. Several new, outstanding GNPs had been hired to work on a contract basis. They were received well in the nursing homes, especially those that had several CC2 members. Fifteen physicians were under contract, six of whom had eleven or more patients. In fact, one physician was caring for 20 patients. Residents seemed positive about their care.

Naomi also described continuing barriers to program expansion, including the restrictive state regulatory environment, limitations of the state nurse practice act, lack of public knowledge and provider experience with managed care, and the general lack of physician involvement in nursing homes.

Linda Nelson, the corporate marketing director, described marketing programs held at area nursing homes to generate "leads." After sponsoring an entertainment event, nursing homes would typically share their lists of residents, to whom information was distributed by mail, and also to their families. She also presented current membership data (see Table 18.1) and referral sources (Table 18.2) for new CC2 members during the current year.

Finally, Jenny described program hospitalization rates and overall financial status. Hospital utilization was reported at 836 admissions and 5,065 days per 1,000 members, with an average length of stay of 6.05 days. All of these levels were higher than for the previous year. The large number of transfers from Healthwise, and the high utilization rates of

Table 18.1 ConstantCaring2 Membership Data Year Three (through December 1)

| | Current Total Membership: 130 | | | |
Quarter	New Members	Transfer In	Transfer Out	Deaths
1st	5	18	2	11
2nd	9	15	3	11
3rd	11	13	3	17
4th (2 months)	15	11	1	9

Table 18.2 ConstantCaring 2 Year Three Referral Sources

Source of New Members Attributed to:	
Physician conversions	67%
Nursing home marketing events	21%
Word of mouth	12%

Table 18.3 ConstantCaring2 Financial Report Year Three Year to Date (through December 1)

Members January 1, this year	97
Members December 1, this year	130
Member months	1,180
Revenue (from Medicare)	$ 925,859
Expenses	
Medical	$1,183,006
Administration/marketing	$ 218,845
Income (loss)	($ 475,992)

these members, were part of the problem. The financial status of the program through November shows a deficit of almost $500,000 (see Table 18.3) for the current year. There was a sense of frustration and desperation on the part of the corporate leaders.

Vigorous discussion ensued about the market for this product and who the customers really were. One member identified a mismatch between marketing efforts and where purchasing decisions are made, and others agreed. Some talked about the changes taking place in the nursing home industry. They focused on the nursing home's evolution toward subacute units, intensive short-term rehabilitation programs, and more specialized longer-term care, especially for seriously cognitively impaired residents. For example, at least 15 percent of area facilities offer dementia care units. Could the CC model develop specialized physician and GNP teams to work on specialized units? All of the residents of a special care unit might be enrolled in ConstantCaring2. This would be especially beneficial to families with limited resources who want quality medical care and quality of life for their loved ones, but who also need to reduce their liability for medical care costs for long-lived Alzheimer's patients.

As the advisory committee discussion continued, other forces affecting nursing home care and CC2's progress in the state were identified: low

Medicaid reimbursement rates; expansion of assisted living facilities and in-home alternatives; a successful, comprehensive Medigap supplemental insurance plan offered in the area; and fear of conflict with the nurse practice act and other state regulatory practices.

Dr. Henry Alpine was introduced at the meeting. He was an experienced internist and geriatrician, recently hired as a full-time medical director at ConstantCaring's corporate headquarters. His responsibilities include establishing critical pathways of care, designing physician and team education seminars, and assisting in physician recruitment. He reported on planned expansion of the CC program into six additional cities over the next three years. The CC model had generated substantial federal interest, and its success at controlling medical costs for the frail elderly was being monitored by the Health Care Financing Administration.

As the luncheon wrapped up, Jenny emphasized that the parent corporation was concerned about continuing financial losses at CC2, and that if membership did not increase quickly, the new site would not survive. As an aside, she mentioned the just completed deal announced in the local newspapers. The parent corporation recently had bought another HMO in the area with 300,000 members, including a very large Medicaid population. She wondered if a relationship with this new, politically savvy partner might assist with CC2 membership development.

In closing, Jenny provided a note of optimism. She reported on a meeting held the previous day with the president of one of the state's nursing home associations. He had recently reviewed the ConstantCaring product and felt it would be excellent, especially for homes that provided a large amount of nonskilled care and needed to upgrade their medical services.

Making the Decisions: Where Does the Program Go?

A week after the meeting, Jenny reviewed the advisory committee's recommendations. Sitting alone in her office on a wintry day, hundreds of miles from the CC2 site, she knew she must do something quickly. After all this time and effort, the program was at risk of closing. She wondered what she could do to save it. There were so many things that could be done, but what were the most critical steps to be taken to keep the program alive?

References

Grace, H. K., L. Kepferle, J. Kress, L. Gaarder, S. McDermott, and S. Jacques. 1988. "Can Geriatric Nurse Practitioners Improve Nursing Home Care?" Final report to W. K. Kellogg Foundation, Boise, ID: Mountain States Health Corporation.

Riverview Residences, Inc.: Growing Pains in Residential Services for Developmentally Disabled Persons

Diane P. S. Shipe

LISA CROCKER had not seen it coming, but in retrospect she thought she should have. Earlier that week, two of the agency's facilities had failed to pass a licensing inspection for the third time. That, plus significant deficiencies at some other facilities, now threatens the continued operation of the entire agency.

Background

Resident Services and Programs

Riverview Residences, Inc., (RRI) is a tax-exempt provider of residential services to individuals with developmental disabilities. The agency provides room and board, supervision, socialization, and habilitation services to its residents. Habilitation refers to structured programs to teach residents to become as independent as possible and includes, for example, activities of daily living, safety education, social interaction skills education, financial management, or sensory awareness training, depending on the resident's functional level and identified individual needs. On weekdays, residents attend an outside program, referred to as a "day program," which might be a paying job, vocational training, a

This is a fictitious case based on the author's experiences in long-term care facility administration.

sheltered workshop, or further habilitation training. The day program is operated by a separate agency.

A resident's overall program must be coordinated and integrated among several providers of services, and this integration is the responsibility of RRI. A resident's needs and problems are identified through an assessment carried out by a staff case manager, a Qualified Mental Retardation Professional (QMRP). A QMRP must have a bachelor's degree in a social services discipline and at least one year experience working with mentally retarded individuals, but this designation does not require licensing. An Individual Habilitation Plan (IHP) is developed by a team of professionals representing the various providers of services, including the day program, county and other social services agencies, transportation, and so on. Depending on the resident's needs, the plan may include residential and day services, transportation, behavioral management and training, various types of therapy, and medical care services. The IHP is structured in the form of needs and problems, long-term goals, short-term goals, and methods. Progress on short-term goals is assessed monthly by the QMRP. The team meets quarterly to review the resident's progress on the goals and to revise the goals and methods as necessary. Each resident receives a full reassessment at least annually. The county social services agency's mental health and mental retardation services unit (MH/MR) has oversight responsibility for each resident's program, and a county caseworker is part of the team. In addition, the resident and a family member or advocate are also part of the team.

Over the years, residents' needs have become much more complex. Those most recently moved into community-based programs tend to be people who are profoundly retarded, who have behavioral or psychiatric problems, or who have significant medical problems. Within the team there are often genuine differences of opinion on how best to meet residents' needs. Occasionally it is very difficult to find an agency willing to accept a particular resident as a client because he or she is seen as having a problematic medical or behavioral history. An agency responds to such a referral by indicating that it is unable to meet the client's needs. In addition to planning, coordinating, and evaluating residents' habilitation programs, case managers are often called upon to handle various crises, particularly those of a behavioral nature, in the homes and with other providers.

RRI operates two types of programs. The first is the community-based residential facility, commonly known as a group home. The second is an intermediate care facility for the mentally retarded (ICF/MR). The residents of the group homes are mostly people who have been moved into the community from large state training centers. These homes have three to six residents. Each home is staffed by at least one direct care staff person afternoons, evenings, nights, early mornings, and weekends. They are operated and regulated under a social model and are licensed by the state department of public welfare. Regulations are written in such a way that RRI holds only one license for all its group homes. Thus, significant deficiencies in one home threaten the licensing status of all the agency's group homes.

The second type of program is the ICF/MR. While the purpose of these facilities is very similar to that of the group homes, they are regulated and licensed by the state Department of Health and are medical model programs, each with an independent license. ICFs/MR are small, generally 8–16 bed, community facilities. Residents of these facilities have extremely complex medical, behavioral, and developmental needs which require nursing and other professional staff support.

ICF/MR residents also have IHPs and habilitation programs. Due to regulatory dictates, these are much more intense than the programs in the group homes. ICF/MR residents must receive "continuous active treatment," which means that some component of their habilitation program must be in progress literally every waking moment. For example, if several residents need assistance in eating, they may not simply sit waiting for a staff person, but should be involved in some activity, such as achieving an aural stimulation goal by listening to music for a specified time each day. Similarly, recreation and social interaction are programmed activities included in the IHP.

Well-designed and implemented habilitation programs have been very successful in teaching people with developmental disabilities the behavioral and daily living skills needed to maximize their levels of independence. Well-trained or experienced case managers, as well as trained, motivated, and caring staff in the homes, are critical to making the habilitation process effective.

RRI's History

RRI was started in 1969 by parents of individuals with developmental disabilities who wanted their children to remain in the community with some independence and not be placed in large state institutions. A number of these families are still active on the Board of Trustees, and their family members are still residents of the programs. James Audell is the sixth executive director of RRI, and has been there for the past four years. The agency has not had good luck with its executive directors; the prior three had short tenures and left under questionable circumstances. Hiring Mr. Audell was something of a coup, since he

Figure 19.1 Riverview Residences, Inc. Program Locations

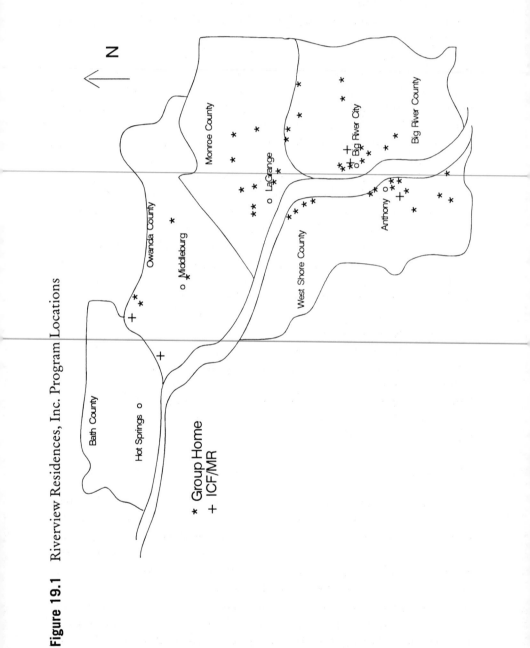

is highly regarded in the professional community for his clinical and administrative expertise.

In the past three years, Mr. Audell led the agency through a period of unprecedented growth, and this occupied almost all of his attention. When he arrived, RRI operated ten group homes and one 20-bed ICF/MR in Big River County. A small agency office was located in Big River City. West Shore County awarded RRI a contract for five new group homes the following year. The agency wrote a successful Certificate of Need (CON) application for a 16-bed ICF/MR to be located there, as well. The second year, additional group home programs were added in West Shore County, a satellite office was located at the West Shore ICF/MR, and RRI won the contract for five group homes in Monroe County. Last year, a CON was awarded for a six-bed ICF/MR in Big River County, four additional group homes were added in both Big River and Monroe Counties, and five were added in West Shore. A satellite office was also added for Monroe County.

Mr. Audell initiated negotiations with Owanda and Bath Counties, which operate a combined mental health and mental retardation social services unit, referred to as a "joinder." Owanda and Bath MH/MR was looking for a residential provider to develop four group homes in Owanda County and two eight-bed ICFs/MR. One ICF/MR was for profoundly retarded individuals with major medical disabilities; the other was for mildly to moderately retarded adolescents with severe behavioral problems. Two more eight-bed ICFs/MR were planned for the following year.

Owanda is an hour's drive from Big River City. Bath's county seat is nearly an hour further up the river. Mr. Audell was successful in winning all of these programs, as well. Because of the distance, a satellite office was set up first in Owanda's county seat, Middleberg. The last of the four group homes opened three months ago; the first two ICFs/MR are to open in another month.

In summary, the agency is presently operating 41 group homes and three ICFs/MR, with two more opening in the immediate future and two more proposed. These facilities provide service to 205 residents (82 in Big River County, 76 in West Shore County, 32 in Monroe County, and 15 in Owanda County). The map in Figure 19.1 shows the locations of each program. Mr. Audell is proud of pointing out RRI is the third largest of 22 residential services providers in the state.

RRI's Financial Situation

The agency is funded almost entirely by Medicaid. Medicaid is a secure, long-term source of funds, although it clearly provides only bare bones

Figure 19.2 Riverview Residences, Inc. Organization Chart

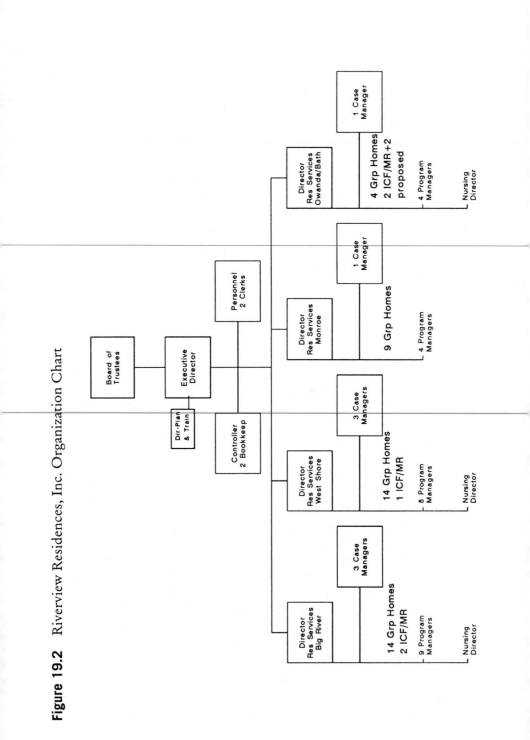

revenues. One of the reasons Mr. Audell gives for promoting the agency's rapid growth is the need to spread administrative overhead costs over a larger number of programs. The agency breaks even or has a one to two percent positive bottom line each year. Cash flow is often a problem. The counties which pay RRI for operating the group homes and the state which administers Medicaid payments for the ICFs/MR make those payments irregularly, based on their budgets and cash availability. The controller has established a short-term line of credit through the bank that helps cover these periods.

Payroll functions and the annual audit are performed under contract by local firms. All other financial functions are handled by RRI staff on two antiquated personal computers. Mr. Audell's secretary has the only other computer, which she uses primarily for word processing. The rest of the staff rely on typewriters and copy machines to do their work.

The group homes and ICFs/MR are rented under three to five year leases from landlords who buy or build the homes as investments. RRI also rents all of its office space. Mr. Audell receives a leased car and cellular phone as part of his compensation.

The agency's assets are extremely limited, but it has successfully used government funding sources to operate needed social services programs, and it has made those funds as productive as possible.

Organization and Staffing

RRI is organized using a geographic model. Figure 19.2 contains the table of organization. Each county where RRI operates has a director of residential services who is responsible for all RRI programs in that county. In addition to Mr. Audell and the four county directors, RRI's senior administration includes (1) the controller, Maria Parodi, CPA (2) the director of personnel, Chondra Washington, and (3) a planner and trainer, Carol LaFalce. Mr. Audell hired all of the senior administrators except Washington, who was promoted from within.

A total of 350 full-time staff are employed, including direct care workers, social workers, nurses, managerial and clerical staff. The majority of employees are direct care staff, called resident advisors (RAs). They receive all of their training from the agency. Topics normally include general information on developmental disabilities, resident rights, fire safety, and relevant procedures and policies, such as documentation, implementation of habilitation programs, medication administration certification for group home staff, implementation of behavior management programs, and self-defense techniques.

Within each county there are case managers who are usually social workers or other professionals qualified as QMRPs. Case managers report to the director of residential services. Regulations limit each case manager's load to 32 residents. RRI generally will not add a case manager position until the maximum caseload is reached.

Program managers (PM) are the first line supervisors at each home and also report to the director; there is one PM for every two group homes. Each ICF/MR has a PM supervising the RA staff, but the charge nurse for an ICF/MR also has an important, although informal, supervisory role. Most PMs are promoted to the position from among the RA staff.

An ICF/MR must have a designated director of nursing, but regulations do not require the position to be full-time for each facility. An individual ICF/MR has nursing, RA, and other professional staff as dictated by residents' needs and regulations.

Clerical staff are centralized in the Big River City office. The satellite offices, at most, have a part-time clerical staff person. Paperwork is mailed to Big River City for typing and then returned. Turnaround takes about a week.

The local economy has been very good for the past five years; however, RRI salaries are low. RAs earn about the same per hour as they could working at a fast food restaurant, and there has been difficulty recruiting RAs, as well as registered nurses and licensed practical nurses. Fortunately, RRI has a very good benefits package, which helps recruitment.

Relationships with County Social Service Agencies

The geographic organizational model is used by RRI for a number of reasons. Physical proximity of program operations is one reason, but the most important is maintaining a good working relationship with each county's social services MH/MR agency. There is a certain amount of ongoing negotiation that takes place with the county's director of MH/MR services relating to resident placement and annual contracts for the group homes.

In addition, the county caseworkers participate in development of IHPs and are extremely influential in decisions regarding a resident's program. The county controls funding for all of a group home resident's services and must agree to finance those services included in the IHP, but not those which are in the residential services contract. The day program and transportation to and from it are routinely financed by the county. Medical and dental care are paid for by Medicaid. Difficulties arise in attempting to coordinate and finance services for a resident with a large number of, or unusual needs, such as for a psychologist, extended therapy and rehabilitation, or specialized adaptive equipment such as an electronic language board for communication.

In the ICFs/MR, by contrast, RRI is responsible for meeting all of a resident's needs from the Medicaid per diem rate received for each resident. The only exceptions are medical and dental services covered under Medicaid, and special education programs for school age children. The ICFs/MR generally have contracts that specify an hourly rate with a physician who acts as medical director; psychologist; physical, occupational, speech, and recreational therapists; and dietitian. The RRI case manager and director of residential services must arrange for and finance any services the resident needs beyond those the facility regularly provides.

County case workers also "monitor" the programs by performing monthly audits of the residents' records. Because of this, each county's MH/MR program demands somewhat different record-keeping of RRI's programs. This is in addition to those records required by the state regulations. The result has been that there are few standard forms and no standardized record systems within the agency. In fact, records may vary even within a county, depending on the demands of county caseworkers.

Overall, the relationships with the county MH/MR units are good in spite of these areas of potential conflict. In Big River County, the agency is well-established and has a good reputation. In Owanda and Bath, the relationship is just being established. There have been some stresses and strains in West Shore, mostly related to differing views on resident needs.

Critical Events

Lisa had worked for RRI since the beginning of February. She had interviewed for a similar position at another residential services provider, but was impressed by Mr. Audell. He was clearly very proud of RRI and he convinced her that there was a lot of potential for professional and personal growth.

Now, in late November, she thought about what had happened since February. She was hired to start the programs in Owanda and Bath counties and had effectively accomplished those objectives. When she was first hired, she remembered being surprised that there was no policy and procedure manual. Memos had been written on various subjects and the executive director's secretary promised to go through her files and make copies of the important ones.

There was also no standardized resident record-keeping system. Lisa had been referred to Joyce, one of the PMs in Big River County, who was reputed to have a good system. After checking out Joyce's system, Lisa found out that the PMs and case managers pretty much organized the records as they chose and made up forms as necessary.

Finally, the training director did not provide the assistance Lisa anticipated and needed. In opening the new group homes, she basically had to hire and train staff with no experience on her own. Carol, the planner and trainer, made it clear that she was following Mr. Audell's orders, and was too busy responding to requests for proposals for new group homes and writing CONs to help out. Carol did the training in areas requiring a certified person; Lisa, her case manager, and program managers did the rest. "Fortunately," Lisa reflected, "the economy in Owanda County is not as good as downriver, and there is nowhere near the turnover among RA staff as is reported there."

Lisa thought the first failed inspection must have occurred about the time she started. Unannounced inspections by licensing surveyors were not usual for the group homes, but they happened occasionally. When it happened, Lisa had not heard about the two homes that had failed. She questioned the directors for West Shore and Monroe Counties, but they said they didn't know anything about it either. The biggest problems were with the habilitation programs:

- IHPs were incomplete based on residents' needs and were poorly developed.
- There were no goals in some areas where residents clearly had needs and no arrangements had been made to meet them.
- Where there were goals, the daily programs either were not being carried out correctly by the RAs or at the specified frequency.
- Documentation in residents' records was lacking for daily program activities and medication administration.

A follow-up inspection of the Walnut Street and Jefferson Street homes had taken place during the summer; no one seems to have heard about the results of this either. Repeat deficiencies are extremely serious, and there were several. A new problem had emerged, too. Monthly menus must be planned which provide residents with a balanced and appealing diet. Apparently residents were eating mostly pizza and fast food for dinner.

In early fall, Mr. Audell brought in a dietitian to plan cycling menus for all of the group homes. That was a big help and a time-saver for the PMs. "It is a big help for me, too, since I don't have to check the menus now. We are not dietitians," thought Lisa. No reason had been given for that action, and beyond that, not much seemed to change. Lisa mused further, "It's an hour's drive to Big River City and I was busy opening new programs. Maybe I just didn't hear what was going on. It certainly would be interesting to know what the board knew about the failed inspections."

The agency's annual licensing survey for the group homes occurs in November. In October, Mr. Audell told the directors what had been happening and stressed the importance of doing well. It wasn't clear what steps were being taken elsewhere, but Lisa knew her programs were in good shape after doing mock surveys of each one. The staff had some experience under their belts. The residents had been in the homes long enough that their needs were understood, and they had made successful transitions from their prior living arrangements. In fact, she had been giving most of her attention to the ICF/MR programs that would open next month.

The outcome that her programs were cited for only one deficiency was little consolation right now. This surveyor had gone through everything with a fine-toothed comb. She had not liked one element of the dental plan form, which was a minor problem. Ironically, it was one of the few forms in agencywide use, so every program was cited on this one. No, what was worse was that problems with the habilitation plans and programs were widespread and showed up in 11 programs in Big River and Monroe Counties. Even worse were questions of falsified records at the Walnut Street and Jefferson Street programs. The Big River County case worker had monitored records two weeks prior to the survey and noted incomplete documentation of carrying out residents' plans. Missing areas had been completed by the time he accompanied the licensing surveyor during the inspection of those programs.

In thinking about the future, Lisa knew the agency could, at best, hope for a three-month provisional license. At the end of that time there would have to be another survey of every group home program. A single serious or repeat deficiency meant the agency would lose its license for all 41 group homes. Technically, loss of the license could be appealed, but Lisa couldn't think of any legitimate or successful grounds on which an appeal could be made.

"This is bound to get to the newspapers and the TV station in Big River City. The residents' families and advocates will have to be told something, and the staff too," Lisa mused. And further, "The county MH/MR agencies will get some really poor publicity out of this. They'll hate that. Controversy is bad in county government. What about their working relationship, which was so new? What would this mean when the contract for the four homes came up for renewal in May?"

The professional staff is already at work preparing for opening the two new ICFs/MR. The RAs will start training in two weeks. Lisa thought more about this situation, "The Department of Public Welfare and the Department of Health surveyors are bound to talk to each other about this. What will they think? What is the status of RRI's other ICFs/MR?

They must have had licensing surveys this year. Should I recommend postponing opening the two new facilities I am responsible for? Financially, can we afford to do that?"

Finally, Lisa got to the most troubling questions. The four Owanda County programs are well-run and effective. The dental plan can easily be changed, and her programs will again pass a licensing survey with flying colors. But, she and her 35 staff members are at the mercy of a lot of other people. What should be her strategy relative to the other directors and their programs? So far no one had been fired. Should she offer to help get those programs in compliance? What will that take? Is it even possible in the available time, given the scope of the problems and the retrospective nature of a licensing survey? She wasn't even sure how or why things had gotten so far out of compliance. Would she have the authority, and frankly, does she want to take on that responsibility? It will mean a lot of time on the road, and her own programs need regular attention too.

She had only talked to Mr. Audell briefly, just long enough to find out the results of the survey and for him to tell her he was calling a meeting of the senior administrators and the board tomorrow at 9:30 a.m.

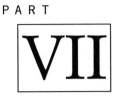

Strategic Planning
and Marketing

Northeast Health Systems:
A Time for Reform

Pamela P. Sawyer

IT WAS A crisp, clear October morning as Nina Price drove north from
Boston on Route 128 toward Beverly, Massachusetts. Her destination
was Northeast Health Systems, Inc./Beverly Hospital. Nina worked as
a health care management consultant for a Boston consulting firm. Her
firm had recently signed a contract with Northeast Health Systems, Inc.
(NHSI), to assist in preparing their response to a federal government
request for proposal (RFP). The RFP (Exhibit 20.1) was for the implementation of a comprehensive health care delivery system. In order to
determine how to advise NHSI, Nina first had to examine the existing
system and area demographics. On the advice of a senior partner in
the firm, she decided to interview six key individuals at NHSI. Along
with the interviews, Nina planned to research the area demographics and
epidemiology.

Northeast Health Systems, Inc./Beverly Hospital

The Beverly Hospital senior management, board of trustees, and medical
staff held a planning retreat in May 1982. During the retreat, the attendees identified the need for corporate restructuring in order to preserve
financial integrity and high-quality patient care services. The corporate
restructuring was established under a parent holding company, Northeast

Real names of people and places have been used in this case.
Prepared under the direction of Paul J. Lanzikos, Simmons College, Boston, MA.

Exhibit 20.1 Summary of the Request for Proposal
Comprehensive Health System for the Older Adult Population

The Secretary of Health and Human Services has been directed by President
Clinton to implement comprehensive health service systems for the older
adult population at a minimum of 12 sites, representing every region of the
country. Following a one-year development period, the Health Care Financing
Administration (HCFA) is to provide payment to these sites on a prepaid
capitated basis for five years for health services currently covered under Medicare,
Medicaid, and supplemental insurance programs.

The objectives of the federal government as they relate to the project are to:

1. Contain health care costs
2. Simplify procedures for obtaining and receiving care
3. Optimize functional capabilities and overall quality of life among the defined
   population.

The primary focus of the comprehensive system is on service delivery reform
through the establishment of integrated health care networks for a targeted
population. The pertinent aspects of the request for proposal (RFP) are listed
below.

Service area: A geographical area, including a senior service facility, where the
target population resides, and where a sufficient number of enrollees reside to
make the system viable.

Targeted beneficiaries: The system will be made available to people aged 65
and over in the target area. The services of the system will be made available to all
persons eligible for Medicare, Medicaid, and supplemental insurance programs.

Services to be provided: The following services must be provided by members
of the comprehensive health care system:

1. Medical care, including primary care physicians and medical/surgical
   specialists
2. Acute hospital care
3. Long-term care, including skilled nursing home care, rehabilitative services,
   adult day health care, homemaker and chore services, home-delivered meals,
   and assisted living arrangements
4. Restorative services, including nursing, home health care, and short-term
   rehabilitative services, both inpatient and outpatient
5. Health prevention and promotion programs, including health clinics and
   screenings, self-help technology, and care giver support
6. Drugs, supplies, and medical equipment.

The RFP stipulates that a five-year contract, containing a negotiated global
budget, will be awarded. The health care system will be responsible for the
coordination of all care and covered services. There must be a commitment by all
providers in the system to serve between 25 percent and 50 percent of the target
population. A data system must be integrated within all the provider components
emphasizing quality care management, financial management, information

Exhibit 20.1 Continued

management, and systems management. The enrolled population will include frail elders in proportion to their presence in the service area. The system will provide services currently covered under Medicare, Medicaid, and supplemental insurance programs. Contracts will be awarded to more than one health care system in the same geographic region, if they fulfill the requirements. Private long-term care may be offered through long-term care or pay-as-you-go.

Health Systems, Inc. This vertically and horizontally integrated system was designed to provide all levels of health care services including acute, long-term, ambulatory, rehabilitative, and home care (Figure 20.1). The attendees also reaffirmed their commitment to programs and services for elders by adding a new senior management position, the vice president for geriatric services.

The focal point of the system is Beverly Hospital, a 234-bed acute care, nonprofit community hospital. It is located approximately 25 miles northeast of Boston on a 38-acre campus in the city of Beverly. Its market service area comprises 22 cities and towns, with a population of 437,227. This is a population decrease of 2.38 percent since the 1980 census (Table 20.1). The hospital is a modern facility offering services such as the state's first freestanding birth center, a regional dialysis center, and the Center for Family Development. Three years ago the hospital added a Level II special care nursery, the North Shore Regional Laser Center, and an additional magnetic resonance imaging (MRI) unit. According to the Massachusetts Health Data Consortium fiscal year (FY) database for that year, the top five clinical subspecialty areas utilized at Beverly were cardiology, obstetrics, Neonatology, general surgery, and orthopedics. The hospital's commitment to the elderly community is evidenced by its Senior Outreach Programs. These include lifeline, informational newsletters (Living Right Along), lecture series, and health promotion clinics.

The principal subsidiaries of Northeast Health Systems, Inc., which demonstrate vertical integration are:

- *Ledgewood Rehabilitation and Skilled Nursing Center* is a 122-bed long-term care and rehabilitation facility located on the campus of Beverly Hospital. It opened in December 1985, and is operated by Ledgewood Health Care Corporation, a sister corporation of NHSI, and the Hillhaven Corporation.
- *The Bay Area Visiting Nurse Association (VNA) Inc.* joined NHSI in 1985. It has provided personalized, high-quality, comprehensive home care to North Shore residents since 1904. According to Judith Thomson, executive director, Bay Area VNA makes over 45,000

Figure 20.1 Northeast Health Systems, Inc.
Corporate Organization Chart

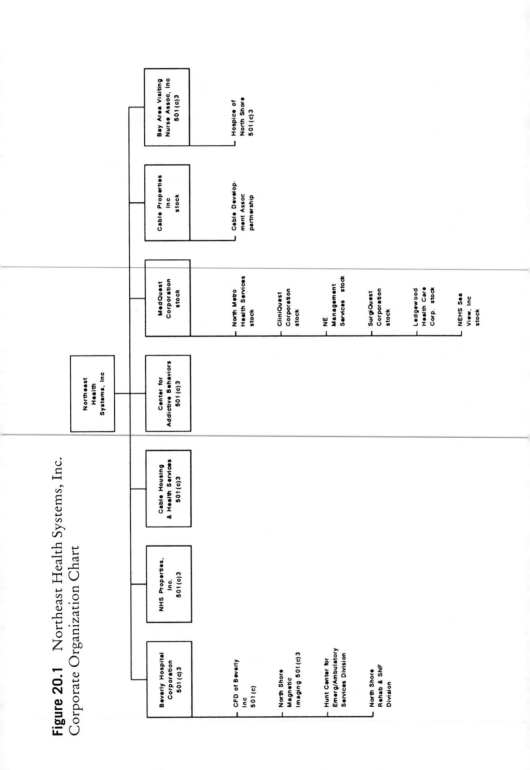

Table 20.1 Beverly Hospital Market Service Area Population Projections

Year	Total Population	0–4 years	5–9	10–14	15–19	20–24	25–29	30–34	35–39	40–44
1970	433,565	35,423	43,261	44,456	38,558	29,589	26,421	22,359	23,923	27,216
1980	423,277	23,755	26,817	34,558	40,150	36,226	33,437	32,118	26,313	21,571
Change	−2.38%	−32.94%	−38.01%	−21.99%	4.13%	22.43%	26.55%	43.65%	9.99%	−20.74%
1990	437,727	30,359	27,315	24,704	27,870	32,103	36,775	38,835	35,965	32,882
Change	3.31%	27.80%	1.86%	−28.78%	−30.59%	−11.38%	9.98%	20.91%	36.68%	52.44%
1995	444,229	27,869	27,676	27,217	27,900	28,312	32,790	36,553	37,300	35,721
Change	1.60%	−8.20%	1.32%	10.17%	0.11%	−11.81%	−10.84%	−5.88%	3.71%	8.63%
2000	451,230	25,378	28,034	29,729	27,933	24,523	28,805	34,273	38,641	38,564
Change	1.58%	−8.94%	1.29%	9.23%	0.12%	−13.38%	−12.15%	−6.24%	3.59%	7.96%

Year	45–49	50–54	55–59	60–64	65–69	70–74	75–79	80–84	85+
1970	27,360	26,092	22,498	19,040	15,095	12,824	9,341	5,934	4,166
1980	22,639	25,134	24,735	21,547	17,656	13,929	9,917	6,961	5,635
Change	−17.26%	−3.67%	9.94%	13.17%	16.97%	8.62%	6.17%	17.31%	35.26%
1990	25,902	20,573	20,445	20,907	19,521	16,234	12,145	8,088	6,604
Change	14.41%	−18.15%	−17.34%	−2.97%	10.56%	16.55%	22.47%	16.19%	17.20%
1995	29,640	25,592	22,415	19,920	18,514	16,594	13,219	8,856	8,131
Change	14.43%	24.40%	9.64%	−4.72%	−5.16%	2.22%	8.84%	9.50%	23.12%
2000	33,375	30,615	24,389	18,932	17,501	16,957	14,295	9,626	9,662
Change	12.60%	19.63%	8.80%	−4.96%	−5.47%	2.19%	8.14%	8.70%	18.83%

home visits per year. It also manages the Spectrum Center, a licensed adult day health program at Cable Gardens. Last year, Bay Area VNA, as a part of a collaborative effort with the Danvers Council on Aging, North Shore Elder Services, and the Hunt Center, opened Spectrum II, a day respite center for people and families coping with Alzheimer's Disease and related disorders.

- *Cable Housing and Health Services Corporation* was established to develop Beverly Hospital's property in Ipswich, Massachusetts. The result was Cable Gardens, a 70-unit elderly congregate housing facility. The $8 million project is a model for mixed income rental housing for frail elders. The Ipswich property is also the site of an emergency room, medical office building, preschool day care center, and the Spectrum II adult day respite program.

- *The Hunt Center for Emergency and Ambulatory Care* in Danvers, Massachusetts, is located on the campus of the former Hunt Memorial Hospital. The Hunt Center has a full-service laboratory, x-ray department, plus outpatient surgery and rehabilitation services. Two years ago, a 60-bed skilled nursing facility opened there. This fills a gap in the continuum of services for patients needing rehabilitation to achieve their maximum level of functioning.

- *The Hospice of the North Shore* merged with Northeast Health Systems four years ago. This Medicare-certified and licensed hospice program offers a full range of services to meet the physical, emotional, and spiritual needs of terminally ill patients and their families.

Northeast Health Systems horizontally integrated by affiliating with the Center for Addictive Behaviors (CAB). CAB offers short- and long-term detoxification on an outpatient basis, methadone maintenance programs, shelter and counseling to addicted women and their children, and peer action groups that work on education and prevention.

North Shore Magnetic Imaging Center is a joint venture with NHSI, AtlantiCare, Addison Gilbert and Salem Hospitals. The Center recently added magnetic resonance angiography services. This procedure allows for noninvasive visualization of blood vessels.

Nina's first scheduled interview that day was with Linda Cragin, the director of geriatrics at NHSI/Beverly Hospital. It was her responsibility to develop programs for the elderly. Her office was located four miles from Beverly Hospital in Danvers, at the Hunt Center. This was Nina's second meeting with Linda. At their first meeting, Linda spent over two hours describing the history and components of NHSI. Linda was eager to show Nina the newly opened day care center just down the hall from her office.

Today's visit was to discuss the RFP and how Linda would respond to it. To Nina's surprise, Linda's office was filled with boxes and stacks of papers everywhere. Nina learned that Linda had taken a new position in Worchester and was scheduled to leave NHSI in a month. Linda felt this new position would "round out" her health care experiences.

Linda began the conversation by stating, "This is going to be a difficult request for proposal to respond to. I've been working on it for two years. The target population, 15,000 to 30,000 people, is a high penetration for this type of project. Marketing and education are going to be very tough. The issue of capacity, particularly in long-term care, is significant. There will have to be relationships with all the area nursing homes. Transportation is also going to be a problem in this area. Public transportation is very limited.

"To manage the overall system, there needs to be an entry point where people are identified with a care manager or primary care physician who provides a coordinating function and identifies the full range of services required. The care manager needs to have a position of authority within the system. He or she must be able to request services, and know what community services are out there and how to access them. The care manager is someone who can advocate for the client and control costs, someone neither from the hospital nor the home health agency.

"Obviously, an information system must be developed. One which has capacity to track a person's medical and functional condition and what it costs to provide the services. It also needs to be user-friendly for providers. We need a financial analysis of our true costs and to track costs as a person moves along the continuum, especially a unit substitution value for each service. We can't track people now in our system. There's no common identifier. We might know what we charge for something, but we don't know what we could have saved if we provided a different mix of services."

In response, Linda noted that the RFP did not address housing issues. If the system succeeds in improving a person's functional abilities, enabling him or her to leave a long-term care facility, where would the person go? There must be some type of housing or housing subsidies. The critical objectives of the RFP, in her opinion, are "to manage people as efficiently and effectively as possible across time, place, and profession."

Before Nina left, Linda rummaged through her boxes to find information she thought might be helpful. Some of the material pertained to the National Chronic Care Consortium (NCCC), of which Beverly Hospital is a member. NCCC is an organization consisting of 14 acute and long-term care providers. The experience, capability, diverse geographic locations, and organizational arrangements of NCCC members allow it to "serve as a national laboratory" for health care reform. Each provider in the consortium is working on developing a geriatric care network that contains a complete continuum of preventive, acute, transitional, and long-term care services in its community.

Nina left The Hunt Center and drove to North Beverly, where she met with Judith Thomson, executive director of the Bay Area Visiting Nurse Association. It was midmorning by the time she arrived, and the office was bustling. It was hard to imagine how the 50 employees got their work done in such a crowded and noisy space. Judith seemed oblivious to the confusion and, after offering Nina a much welcomed cup of coffee, proceeded to discuss the RFP. Although she had scheduled one an hour, this interview lasted over two.

Judith said, "I think it's better to look at the RFP from the perspective of community versus acute care. Unfortunately, people still see the hospital as the critical piece. I'm not so sure that's true anymore. A patient may not necessarily have to go to the hospital for every medical encounter. The physician would be pivotal, but the system should be managed by a care management entity. The entity would be the liaison with all of the other providers in the system.

"To track a person through the continuum of care, a computer database system is needed. There would be multiple entry points into the system, and not everyone will need care management. The computer system would have to identify a person as to whether they received services or not.

"Ethical and moral dilemmas need to be considered. Routinely, these issues deal with clients who have cognitive impairment, no family support, are at constant risk, and the funds available to provide them with health and support services are limited.

"To make a system like this work will take a lot of education. Except for the upper management team, the providers in NHSI don't view it as a real system. Physicians need to be educated to all the services within the system. Elders and their families are not always aware of what health care options are available to them, and therefore rely on the physician to help them. This education could be presented in a marketing form. I feel the customers of the system, physicians and elders, would respond to this mode of education."

Judith saw the financial requirements of the RFP as the most difficult area to determine. She used many VNA client cases as examples of how she would respond to the RFP. She concluded by saying, "I very strongly believe we're going to have to go to something like this, and I don't mind sharing the risk. Just give me the parameters so that we can do it well and make sure that all of the pieces are there."

Nina also tried to obtain a clearer description of the communities served by NHSI. The greater North Shore area, the primary market service area, was characterized by the following demographics:

- The communities ranged from rural to light industrial suburban.
- According to the 1990 census, the largest growth over the past ten years has been in the population over 65 years of age, increasing from 12.8 percent to 15 percent. This cohort is projected to continue to increase, especially the group over 85 years-old. The region's population of elderly exceeds the national average (15 percent versus 11.8 percent).
- The region has a shortage of nursing home beds, a lower bed to population ratio than the state (56.1 beds per 1,000 compared to 86.9 beds per 1,000). The number of beds is projected to be under 30 per 1,000 beds next year, the lowest ratio in the state.
- Admitting diagnoses at Beverly Hospital indicate disease rates consistent with national projections for comparable populations. The only exception is a greater than normal incidence of Lyme disease in one area.
- The elderly population in the area has a higher than the national average income level.

The next round of interviews took Nina to the administrative offices of Beverly Hospital where she spent time with Brad Silsby, vice president of strategic planning. Brad's forte was statistical data, but a recent personal experience with community-based home care had greatly increased his desire to develop an integrated health system. Brad said:

"I don't think we've envisioned all of the better ways we can take care of patients. It would be useful to have a geriatrician on the senior management staff. Physicians are faced with many complex problems. A geriatrician could act as a consultant to all the providers in the system. The RFP will require all the providers to optimize the functional capabilities of the system's enrollees. Our philosophy is to rehabilitate and promote independence in our clients, not just to maintain them.

"In the North Shore area we have a relatively affluent, highly educated elderly population. The physicians know that various agencies exist, but don't have time to spend in the home setting. The hybrid care management entity created from the hospital and community that manages the overall system would be responsible for education and marketing. After marketing the system to physicians, they, in turn, would market the services to their patients."

The RFP calls for a negotiated global budget. Brad described a fairly complicated model to accomplish this based on the number of enrollees, utilization of services, and projected cost. Brad was confident that NHSI had the data and ability to comply with this request.

A few doors down from Brad's office was the office of Bob Fanning, president of Beverly Hospital. As Nina waited for the interview she noticed numerous awards on display: they were testimony to his achievements as an exemplary leader in the health care arena. Over the past 11 years, he had demonstrated his commitment to the patients, employees, and corporate mission of NHSI and Beverly Hospital (Exhibit 20.2).

Bob began the interview by stating that the corporate restructuring and vertical integration that had begun in 1982 was partly designed to meet a future "capitation model" of reimbursement. He felt, therefore, that NHSI was in a good position to reply to the RFP.

"The good news is we already have a continuum of care in place. The buzz word of today is 'managed competition.' We are setting up a physician-hospital organization (PHO) that will monitor and manage patients on a continuum of care basis. The PHO will develop care guidelines for care management. A comprehensive health care delivery system like this has to be physician-driven. Physicians need to get involved in a system of reimbursement that rewards them for managing care, as opposed to delivering care. we will have to learn the ins and outs of risk contracting.

Nina asked Bob how the physicians would access the support services in the community. Bob explained that it would have to be done through the discharge planning process. According to Bob, though, the system doesn't work like that now. "It doesn't always work because we don't have the commitment to make it work. Our social services departments work Monday through Friday, nursing homes traditionally haven't admitted patients on the weekend, and home health agencies have only just started to admit and service patients over the weekend. You need a czar who says that this is the way its going to be. I think managed care is going to make all that easier."

The continuum has been operating for over five years and the people who operate it share a common work ethic and ability to communicate with each other. NHSI is exploring the possibility of developing medically assisted housing. This will fill a niche in the existing system. As to an information for a comprehensive system like this, "no one in the industry has one," according to Bob. Finally, he felt it was very important that the system have "a name" which gave it recognition in the health care market place.

A few days later Nina was back at Beverly Hospital visiting Beth

Exhibit 20.2 Corporate Mission Statement for Northeast Health Systems, Inc.

The mission of Northeast Health Systems, Inc., (the Corporation), is to encourage and promote health services for the greater North Shore community and to stimulate the development of health-related and other services, with the overall purpose of contributing to and advancing the health and well-being of the community without restriction to race, color, creed, national origin, or ability to pay. The objectives of the Corporation shall include, but are not limited to the following:

a. *Acute and Ambulatory Care.* To encourage and foster a comprehensive range of inpatient and outpatient health care services, including prevention, diagnosis, treatment, restoration, rehabilitation, etc., to enable patients to lead healthy productive lives.

b. *Health Promotion.* To participate in community and regional activities having as their purpose the maintenance of health and the prevention of illness and injury, and to seek innovative means to improve the effectiveness and efficiency of the delivery of health care services.

c. *Long-term Care.* To promote and encourage the development of programs and services for the elderly and the chronically and terminally ill in various settings which maximize independent functioning, achieve the greatest degree of comfort and dignity, and involve family and friends in the caring process.

d. *Comprehensive System.* To develop and oversee a comprehensive health care system which facilitates access to needed health care services, and to the provision of those services, in a coordinated manner.

e. *Related and Supportive.* To stimulate the development of other services or activities which may benefit the community at large, while maintaining the viability of the corporation.

f. *Education and Research.* To develop and advance such educational, scientific research, and scholarly activities related to health care and to the promotion and maintenance of good health as deemed feasible and appropriate.

g. *Financial Strength.* To encourage and foster financial and operational stability among all aspects of the system.

Dimitruk, the director of the Senior Outreach Program. Beth was clearly an advocate for elders in the community. Her expertise was in coordinating the senior programs managing the lifeline program, and providing the community with information. Detailed responses to an RFP were foreign to her. She envisioned a physician from the hospital overseeing the whole operation. When asked if the medical staff knew what's in the community and how to access services for their clients she replied:

"They haven't a clue as to what's available in the community. I really think they want to be educated, because it's so difficult treating elders. They have such diverse needs. The needs of an active 65-year-old are different from an 85-year-old with multiple health problems. Likewise, the needs of Betty Tuff, the editor of our newsletter, who's 85 and just bought her own computer, are different from both. It's very difficult to target the needs of this population."

Nina knew it was time to speak with a member of the medical staff. The medical staff had 373 members representing all specialties. Nina scheduled an interview with Dr. Herbert Bistrong, president of Beverly Hospital Medical Staff. He graciously agreed to meet her in the early morning on his day off. Dr. Bistrong said, "I think the time has come for managed care. Good quality medical care doesn't have to be expensive. At NHSI we know how to control costs. We closely monitor lengths of stay and what it costs for a patient to stay in the hospital. I don't see why a risk sharing system like this can't be done. A system like this requires that the gatekeeper be the primary care physician, family practitioner, or internist. I don't mean to exclude the paraprofessional people who work at keeping the patient out of the hospital. There needs to be a partnership. The physician does not have to make all the decisions, but has to be the person who coordinates this. He or she really controls the high end of the cost in this situation. Nobody else can make those kinds of decisions."

Dr. Bistrong described how to educate physicians to the comprehensive care system and its community services: "A capitated rate would be the incentive. You affect his bottom line. There is nothing more educational than saving money. We're crisis-oriented. It's part of our training. I think physicians need to be brought up to speed about what the resources are and how to use them expeditiously for their patients. It is overwhelming today. Everybody is overloaded and working as hard as they can. Physicians see 20, 30, sometimes 40 patients a day, plus run their offices and interface with Medicare and other payers. The thrust of a capitated system is to keep people out of the hospital. To share in the profitability, physicians will be driven to learn what's in the community.

"From the physician's standpoint, if you have capitation, this doesn't have to mean rationing health care. I think what it does is drive the physician to look very closely at delivering cost-effective care. There's a lot to be cut out of the existing system in the way of inefficiencies. You can make the system run much, much better and have quality care."

Dr. Bistrong concluded the interview by stating that NHSI had all the pieces, except they didn't "exactly mesh with each other." As Nina walked out of the medical library toward the elevators, she wondered how she was going to find a way to respond to the RFP and incorporate the widely varying suggestions she had received to date. Questions stuck in her mind:

- Did the system have the capacity to respond to the RFP?
- Were the present service organizations capable of responding to the needs of the defined population, or would the organization have to change?
- How could this fragmented system be unified?
- Who would manage the comprehensive system?
- Who would be the cornerstone provider of the continuum of care?
- How could an integrated information system be developed within budgetary constraints?

21

Ocean Point Retirement Community: The Viability of a Continuing Care Retirement Community

Arnold M. Possick and Robert C. Myrtle

Statement of the Problem

TWO YEARS ago, Ocean Point Retirement Community (OPRC), a not-for-profit continuing care retirement community with a long and distinguished record of serving the needs of elderly people, received notice from the Portwell city government that its facilities did not meet current local safety codes. The city had decided to more strictly enforce these building regulations because the area had been experiencing frequent seismic activity. The main building of OPRC was developed as a resort hotel in 1929, with cottages and a skilled nursing facility having been added over the years. To comply with the seismic safety code, OPRC would need substantial and costly renovation of its building structures. Such renovation, however, would still leave it with noncompetitive living units and amenities in today's and future markets. Ocean Point Retirement Community, together with its parent corporation, must present a plan to the Portwell city government within the next 120 days. Today it is May 1.

North Valley Homes—The Parent Corporation

North Valley Homes (NVH) is the parent corporation for three continuing care retirement communities, one of which is OPRC, and a

This case is based on a real organization, but names of people and places have been changed to assure anonymity.

freestanding skilled nursing facility. It manages, but does not own, three other retirement communities (see Figure 21.1, map of Facility Locations). Honest, open communication between NVH and its owned properties is the norm. Major strategic decisions for the owned properties are made by the NVH Board of Directors and by the corporate executive staff; the individual facilities do not have their own boards of directors. North Valley Homes is a not-for-profit, religiously sponsored organization (see Figure 21.2, Organization Chart).

Figure 21.1   North Valley Homes

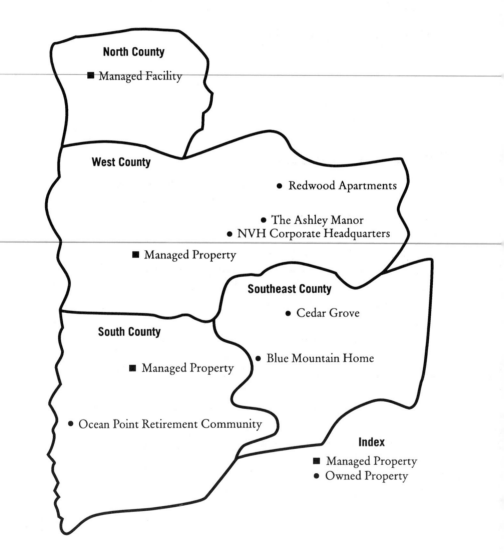

Figure 21.2 North Valley Homes Organization Chart

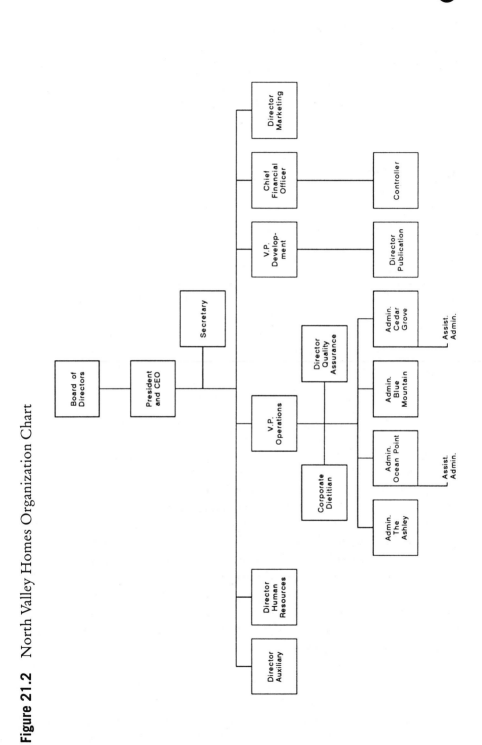

Developmental History of NVH

North Valley Homes was incorporated in 1943 as part of the Social Ministry of America. Its sole purpose was to serve the needs of the elderly. North Valley Homes became the first and only organization specifically serving the elderly in Arlington, West County when in 1944 it purchased land and buildings providing living units for approximately 25 residents. Over the years, new structures were added to the facility that became known as The Ashley Manor (see Exhibit 21.1). By 1965, units for a maximum of 150 residents and a skilled nursing facility for 70 residents had been completed.

In 1960, NVH acquired OPRC, which formerly was owned by the Ministry of South County, representing approximately 100 congregations, at no cost, by transfer of title. Ocean Point Retirement Community had been converted from a resort hotel to a retirement home in 1954, accommodating a maximum of 130 residents (see Exhibit 21.2). A skilled nursing facility for 59 residents was completed across the street from the main building in 1972.

Another property was acquired in 1961 known as Redwood Apartments in Palmdale, West County. This facility, containing apartments for independent living, was built in 1959 by Redwood Homes, Inc. North Valley Homes sold the property in February of this year. The publicly stated reason was that the sale would allow NVH to focus on its continuing care retirement community campuses and on the management of large non-NVH-owned senior apartment complexes.

In 1971, a well-established retirement community in Acton, Southeast County joined NVH. Now known as Cedar Grove, this ten-acre campus includes residential care facilities for over 175 persons, and two years ago completed the construction of a state-of-the-art 99-bed skilled nursing facility (Exhibit 21.3). A former 33-bed skilled nursing facility was converted to additional assisted living accommodations.

As testimony to the fine quality of care offered at the campuses, NVH was one of the first multifacility organizations to earn accreditation for each of its owned continuing care retirement campuses by the Continuing Care Accreditation Commission. Accreditation is an independent assurance of quality beyond the required state licenses for retirement homes and nursing facilities.

Blue Mountain Home, on the verge of bankruptcy, merged with NVH in 1986. Located in Newbury, Southeast County, Blue Mountain began operations in 1958, and is licensed to provide care for 75 persons in its residential section, which includes a nonambulatory assisted living wing (Exhibit 21.4). A skilled nursing facility was opened in 1974, offering several levels of care to 120 residents.

Exhibit 21.1   The Ashley Manor, Arlington, West County

The Ashley Manor is the original home of North Valley Homes. The campus is centrally located on 10 acres of prime hillside, close to freeways and downtown shopping.

Residential care apartments		
	10 Cottages	
	72 Single	333 sq. ft.
	33 Semi-suites	378 sq. ft.
	14 Two-room apartments	549 sq. ft.
	8 Conversions	549 sq. ft.
Total	137	

Personal services: Full programs on A and E levels of residential building

Assisted living apartments	10 Shared (20 beds)

Skilled nursing beds		
	2 Private beds	
	30 Semi-private beds	
	18 Beds (3 bedrooms)	
Total	23 (50 beds)	

Rates

Residential	Accommodation Fee	Monthly Fee	Monthly + Entrance Fee	Monthly Fee
Single	$ 42,000	$ 895	$2,500	$1,690
Semi	49,000	1,010	2,500	1,830
2-room	59,000	1,165	2,500	2,160
Conversion	69,500	1,165	2,500	2,160
Cottages	88,000	1,245	2,500	2,880
Additional person		400		

Personal services (residential) full package: $500 plus room rate

Assisted living: Standard: $1,885   Deluxe: $1,945
Direct admits pay $2,500 entrance fee, $2,025 monthly

Skilled nursing: Private: $115 day, Semi: $102 day, 3-Bed: $90 day
($71.15 day, Medicaid reimbursement)

Current Resident Profile (includes SNF)
Average age is 85 years
Average age of all current residents at entry was 79 years
144 female; 32 male;
171 Anglo; 3 Hispanic; 2 Asian

In 1977, a new division of NVH was formed to provide consultation, training, management, and research services to outside organizations. The division, called North Valley Management Services, manages a government-subsidized independent living, low-cost housing program for approximately 135 elderly deaf people located in Lebec City, West

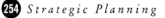

Exhibit 21.2 Ocean Point Retirement Community, Portwell, South County

Residential care apartments	47	Studio apartments
	3	Semi-suite apartments
	33	One-bedroom apartments
	_5	Two-bedroom apartments
Total	88	(18 in cottages; 70 in main building)
Assisted living apartments	9	Studio apartments
	1	Semi-suite (2 beds)
	_1	Suite (2 beds)
Total	11	Rooms, 13 beds
Skilled nursing beds	2	Private beds
	36	Semi-private beds
	21	Beds in three-bed units
Total	59	Beds

Rates

Residential	Accommodation Fee	Monthly Fee
Single	$36,000–$42,000	$ 940
1-Bedroom	$66,000–$80,000	1,220
2-Bedroom	$77,000–$95,000	1,600

	Monthly + Entrance Fee	Monthly Fee
Assisted living	$2,500	$1,800–$2,100
Skilled nursing	$98–$115 per day (Medicaid reimbursement—$73.84/day)	

Current Resident Profile
Current occupancy: Residential: 92; Assisted living: 13
Average age is 85.8 years (61 to 101)
Average age of current residents at time of admission is 79
13% male; 87% female; 8% couples
55% previously lived within a 20-mile radius of OPRC
12% previously lived out of state
46% had annual income of $20,000 and above
100% Caucasian

County. It also manages two other senior developments, one in North County, the other in South County. North Valley Homes now serves close to 1,500 older persons in eight cities. Seven hundred employees care for the residents of its continuing care retirement communities, senior housing developments, and skilled nursing facilities.

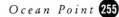

Exhibit 21.3   Cedar Grove, Acton, Southeast County

Residential care apartments	45	Studio apartments
	4	Semi-suite apartments
	29	Suites
	29	One-bedroom apartments
	_8_	Three-bedroom cottages
Total units	115	

Assisted living apartments	28	Private units
	6	Beds in semi-private rooms
	_14_	Beds in two-room suites
Total	48	Beds

Skilled nursing beds	17	Private beds
	_18_	Semi-private beds
Total	99	Beds

Rates

Residential	Accommodation Fee	Monthly Fee
Single	$ 37,700–$40,000	$1,690
Semi-suite	43,800	1,830
1-Bedroom cottage or suite	55,500–68,000	2,160
2-Bedroom cottage	104,500–105,000	2,880

Assisted Living	Monthly + Entrance Fee	Monthly Fee
Shared room & shared bath	$2,500	$1,785
Suite w/private bath	2,500	2,960

Skilled Nursing
Semi-private—$120/day; Parlor suite—$174/day; Max. care unit—$500/day;
($73.50 Medicaid reimbursement)

Current Resident Profile
Average age is 81.6 years;
Average age of existing residents at admission was 80.6 years.
28 males; 105 females; 8% couples
132 Caucasians; 1 Asian

Management of NVH

North Valley Homes, like other continuing care retirement communities, entered a new era of the long-term care industry in the past few years. For over 30 years, NVH was led by William Schaumann, a charismatic man with a vision and an ironclad will. His autocratic style drew many loyal

Exhibit 21.4 Blue Mountain Home, Newbury, Southeast County

Assisted living apartments	50	single apartments with private baths
	6	suites
	6	studios
	4	2-bathroom singles (can be converted)
Total	62	units
Skilled nursing beds	96	private beds (40 beds in secured wing)
	24	semi-private beds
Total	120	beds

Additional Services
Outpatient clinics for speech, occupational and physical therapy
Provide meals for "Meals on Wheels": 31,200 per year, Monday–Friday
Provide meals for "Meals with a Friend": 6,240 per year
Provide meals for child day care: 14,300 per year

Rates
Assisted living: Single: $1,280–$2,547 (reduced fee if require less care)

Skilled nursing: Private: $135 per day (Medicaid reimbursement—$68.81 per day)

Current Resident Profile
Average age is 89
Average age at admission was 85
January of current year, average daily census: 115 SNF; 36 assisted living
Number of admissions last year: 51 SNF; 13 assisted living
Number of admissions, Jan–Mar of current year: 8 SNF; 8 assisted living
Number of deaths last year: 42 SNF; 3 assisted living
Admissions from current year and last year:
68% from within 10-mile radius of Blue Mountain; 39% from town of Newbury
149 Residents are Anglo, 2 Hispanic
9% are male (14); 91% are female (137)

administrators to his staff, who typically served for decades. The board of directors was an inactive body simply rubber stamping Schaumann's ideas. North Valley Homes flourished under these conditions.

Until the late 1980s, long-term care facilities were fully occupied, often with waiting lists. North Valley Homes lacked a marketing department, and did not need one. Budgeting was more a formality than an essential tool; NVH always enjoyed a healthy profit margin. The management of NVH failed to recognize changing demographics and competitive trends in the field (such as room size). By the late 1980s, problems were surfacing at NVH, problems which have continued to the present. The current occupancy rate of NVH retirement communities is 86 percent with no waiting lists, and the past three years have brought substantial and increasing operational losses.

William Schaumann retired three years ago, followed by his entire management team. The new president/CEO of NVH, George Putnam, is a dynamic leader, well-schooled in modern management techniques. In two years he has built a top management team and an active Board of Directors whose members understand the challenges facing NVH. There are now professional marketing departments at NVH and at each of the owned campuses; there are standing committees and task forces to deal with issues proactively; professionally accepted techniques of financial management are used; outside expertise is hired when needed for specific projects, such as an assessment of OPRC's redevelopment possibilities; and difficult management decisions are made and implemented, such as the current freeze on salaries and wages. The NVH board and executive staff are developing a new strategic long-range plan to replace the current one, which is over ten years old.

Putnam's vision for NVH in the year 2001 was expressed at an administrative staff retreat a few years ago, "North Valley Homes' primary identity as an organization providing residential services for those who are aging will have shifted. The identity will be one of an organization with broad expertise in housing, gerontology, and diverse services including education, consultation, and direct care, even as it retains a specific expertise in residential continuums. . . . Our services will be diversified with a large community-based component, . . . we will participate in joint ventures . . . NVH will have entered the ancillary service market to provide durable medical equipment and pharmaceutical services . . . NVH will be recognized for its adaptability and creativity in the midst of change."

Challenges Facing NVH

Increased Debt with Reduced Cash Reserves

The acquisition of Blue Mountain Home four years ago increased NVH's long-term debt by over $6 million. North Valley Homes refinanced the property, enabling it to pay holders of outstanding Blue Mountain notes the full value of their investment (most note holders were church members). This left NVH, however, with a debt exceeding the market value of the property. The financial condition of NVH was further worsened by the construction of a 99-bed skilled nursing facility (SNF) on their Cedar Grove campus. The building project was poorly managed, yielding costly delays in construction and expensive "add-ons." By the time construction was completed two years ago, cost overruns at this state-of-the-art facility were approximately $4.5 million, reducing cash reserves by that amount. Debt payments rose from $300,000 four years ago to $1,800,000 last year.

Increased Charitable Care Expenses

In the past three years, the annual cost of charitable care at NVH increased by more than $3 million, from $874,000 to $3,923,000. One factor behind this trend is the increasing average age of residents entering the facilities. Last year the age at entry averaged in the high 70s or low 80s, while ten years earlier it had been in the mid-70s. The increase in age is accompanied by greater frailty among entering residents and diminished personal resources. This trend exacerbated increasing divestment of assets into family trusts in order to be eligible for Medicaid. As a result, residents exhaust their personal resources more quickly, after which Medicaid becomes the payer source for their care. The cost of charitable care rose at NVH because Medicaid reimbursement does not cover the actual cost of care, the difference being about $1,300 per month for each Medicaid resident.

Charitable care occurs more often in the skilled nursing facilities of continuing care retirement communities (CCRCs) than in their assisted living or independent living components. North Valley Homes' skilled nursing capacity grew by 230 percent, from 142 to 328 beds, with the purchase of Blue Mountain Home and the expanded skilled nursing facility at Cedar Grove. By last year, the percentage of NVH's total income coming from Medicaid had risen to 25 percent, from 8 percent three years earlier.

Increased Competition

The facilities owned and operated by NVH faced a dramatic increase in competition during the mid-1980s to the early 1990s. The in-depth examination of OPRC's competitive market described later in this case serves to illustrate many of the competitive issues confronting OPRC and the other campuses.

Operational Losses

One of NVH's most significant financial issues is its mounting operating deficit. Historically, the organization covered its deficit by tapping its Endowment Fund income—the Fund had a $4.9 million balance last year (see Exhibit 21.5). The deficit trend first surfaced five years ago when there was an operational gain of only $16,168. Losses were $688,734 three years ago, $1,646,038 two years ago, and $1,070,995 last year (see Exhibit

21.6) for a three-year total of $3,405,767. To understand the problem, it is helpful to examine the change in payer mix at the health centers. In the past four years, SNF revenue has doubled as a source of revenue, and a growing share is derived from Medicaid (see Exhibit 21.7).

In order to eliminate its operating deficit, NVH must decrease reliance on SNFs and increase revenue from residential and assisted living, both in dollar amounts and in terms of percentage of total revenue. North Valley Homes has recently implemented a three-year plan to achieve a five percent (gross) operational surplus. The plan calls for a $400,000 operating deficit this year, breaking even next year, and a 5 percent (gross) surplus in two years.

Another factor responsible for the operating losses is the fairly high average vacancy rate of the past few years. As of April 15 of this year, 75 of 340 residential units were vacant, 23 of 143 assisted living units, and 14 of 328 beds in skilled nursing were empty (see Table 21.1). Two additional factors adding to NVH's operational losses have been escalating worker compensation expenses and health care costs.

Aging Buildings and Unfunded Depreciation

Before this year, NVH had never funded its depreciation in part or in total. Reserves were largely spent on Cedar Grove's cost over-runs. Even worse, for decades accommodation fees have been required for operations, rather than retained for capital expenses. All NVH campuses have deferred maintenance and renovation expenses. Ocean Point Retirement Community faces $1.2 to $1.4 million in seismic compliance work, exclusive of facilities upgrading.

The organization only began funding depreciation this year. It budgeted capital expenses at a projected 50 percent of depreciation, which is expected to provide adequate short-term financial support for plant operations and maintenance. In addition, NVH is working with a consulting firm to do demographic and marketing studies of the individual campuses to determine their long-term economic viability, and to determine future capital and maintenance projects.

Ocean Point Retirement Community

The Facility

Ocean Point Retirement Community consists of 88 residential units, 11 assisted living units, and a 59-bed skilled nursing facility adjacent to the ocean. Fifty of the 88 residential units are studio and semi-suite apartments. Of the remaining residential units, 33 are one-bedroom

Text continues on page 265

Exhibit 21.5 North Valley Homes Combined Statements of Changes in Fund Balances
(years ended December 31, last year and two years ago)

	Annuity Fund	Capital Improvement	Quasi-Endowment Fund	General Fund	Total
Restated fund balances—December 31, 3 years ago	$ 163,314	$19,738	$3,863,976	$6,755,232	$10,802,260
Funds Received					
Gifts and contributions	28,995	35,989	630,938	260,297	956,219
Interest and dividends	40,665	1,320	260,779	242,721	545,485
Loss on sale of assets	(3,731)	—	—	(16,891)	(20,622)
Expenses and other	(93,552)	7,646	—	(58,157)	(144,063)
Fund transfers	—	—	(75,048)	75,048	—
Excess of operating expenses over operating revenues of general fund	—	—	—	(1,646,038)	(1,646,038)
Fund balances—December 31, 2 years ago	135,691	64,693	4,680,645	5,612,212	10,493,241
Funds Received					
Gifts and contributions	237,641	—	232,384	274,051	744,076
Interest and dividends	48,296	—	237,962	119,068	405,326
Gain (loss) on sale of assets	15,174	—	189,723	(10,089)	194,808
Expenses and other	(127,031)	—	(41,267)	—	(168,298)
Fund transfers	—	(64,693)	(398,841)	463,534	—
Excess of operating expenses over operating revenues of general fund	—	—	—	(1,070,995)	(1,070,995)
Fund balances—December 31, last year	$ 309,771	—	$4,900,606	$5,387,781	$10,598,158

Exhibit 21.6 North Valley Homes Combined Statement of Revenues and Expenses
(year ended December 31, last year)

	Ashley Manor	Ocean Point	Blue Mountain	Cedar Grove	Four Campus Total
Operating Revenues					
Net resident and patient service revenues	$3,447,044	$3,038,857	$5,042,527	$5,343,665	$16,872,093
Amortization of accommodation fees	434,539	292,192	—	416,518	1,143,249
Change in estimated obligation to provide future services,					
in excess of	205,981	(590,576)	232,014	87,400	(65,181)
Other	65,184	118,226	265,087	149,584	598,081
Total operating revenues	4,152,748	2,858,699	5,539,628	5,997,167	18,548,242
Operating Expenses					
Medical services	1,091,190	1,190,339	2,333,430	1,803,419	6,418,378
Plant facility cost	483,813	347,209	525,160	572,651	1,928,833
Housekeeping and laundry	253,261	256,134	295,745	355,431	1,160,571
Dietary	944,615	917,039	859,832	997,262	3,718,748
Resident services and activities	104,217	101,914	240,826	230,964	677,921
Administration	626,454	786,622	589,435	1,023,377	3,025,888
Interest	55,504	67,412	575,158	624,750	1,322,824
Depreciation and amortization	197,848	175,974	329,780	469,159	1,172,761
Other	44,129	22,662	73,411	74,024	214,226
Total operating expenses	3,801,031	3,865,305	5,822,777	6,151,037	19,640,150
Excess of operating revenues over operating expenses	$ 351,717	($1,006,606)	($ 283,149)	($ 153,870)	($ 1,091,908)

Continued

Exhibit 21.6 Continued

	Redwood Apartments	NV Management Services	The Volunteer Auxiliary	Eliminations	General Fund Total
Operating Revenues					
Net resident & patient service revenues	$191,735	—	—	($191,735)	$16,872,093
Amortization of accommodation fees	—	—	—		1,143,249
Change in estimated obligation to provide future services, in excess of amount received or to be received					(65,181)
Other	14,412	178,883	211,407	(404,702)	598,081
Total operating revenues	206,147	178,883	211,407	(596,437)	18,548,242
Operating Expenses					
Medical services					6,418,378
Plant facility cost	60,132			(60,132)	1,928,833
Housekeeping and laundry					1,160,571
Dietary					3,718,748
Resident services and activities					677,921
Administration	65,550	62,583		(209,438)	2,944,583
Interest				(20,914)	1,301,910
Depreciation and amortization	19,001			62,305	1,254,067
Other	3,127		203,737	(206,864)	214,226
Total operating expenses	147,810	62,583	203,737	(435,043)	19,619,237
Excess of operating revenues over operating expenses	$ 58,337	$116,300	$ 7,670	($161,394)	($ 1,070,995)

Continued

Exhibit 21.6 Continued

North Valley Homes
Combined Statements of Revenues and Expenses
Last Year, Two Years Ago

	Last Year	Two Years Ago
Operating Revenues		
Net resident and patient service revenues	$16,872,093	$16,101,957
Amortization of accommodation fees	1,143,249	946,276
Change in estimated obligation to provide future services in excess of amounts received or to be received	(65,181)	228,644
Other	598,081	497,325
Total operating revenues	18,548,242	17,774,202
Operating Expenses		
Medical services	6,418,378	6,129,322
Plant facility cost	1,928,833	1,955,387
Housekeeping and laundry	1,160,571	1,272,813
Dietary	3,718,748	3,752,893
Resident services and activities	677,921	486,101
Administration	2,944,583	3,003,794
Depreciation and amortization	1,254,067	1,197,590
Interest expense	1,301,910	1,190,174
Other	214,226	432,166
Total operating expenses	19,619,237	19,420,240
Excess of operating expenses over operating revenues	(1,070,995)	(1,646,038)
Nonoperating Revenues		
General fund	383,030	503,018
Board-designated funds	660,069	891,717
Donor-restricted funds	301,111	106,969
Total nonoperating revenues	1,344,210	1,501,704
Nonoperating Expenses		
Board-designated funds	41,267	75,048
Donor-restricted funds	127,031	89,637
Total nonoperating expenses	168,298	164,685
Excess of (expenses over revenues) revenues over expenses	$ 104,917	($ 309,019)

Continued

Exhibit 21.6 Continued

North Valley Homes
Combined Balance Sheets

December 31, Last Year and Two Years Ago	Last Year	Two Years Ago
Current Assets		
Cash	$ 574,804	$ 872,669
Investments	44,918	242,834
Accounts and notes receivable	1,513,181	1,093,579
Prepaid and other assets	327,598	351,600
Total current assets	2,460,501	2,560,682
Property and equipment, net	26,837,478	27,776,070
Assets held for sale	229,840	—
Restricted cash	1,963,347	1,998,249
Restricted and Board-designated investments	5,433,704	5,432,275
Other assets	35,946	61,004
Total assets	$36,960,816	$37,828,280
Liabilities and Fund Balances		
Current liabilities		
Accounts payable and accrued expenses	$ 1,221,783	1,300,066
Current portion of long-term debt	357,178	938,352
Deposits held in trust	85,400	227,900
Total current liabilities	1,664,361	2,466,318
Long-term debt, less current portion	15,275,380	15,611,654
Estimated obligation to provide future services, in excess of amounts received or to be received	959,231	894,050
Annuities payable	701,994	613,270
Other accrued liabilities	2,153,851	1,737,701
Refundable accommodation fees	1,251,000	1,794,000
Deferred revenue from accommodation fees	4,356,841	4,218,046
Total	26,362,658	27,335,039
Commitments and Contingencies		
Fund balances		
General fund	5,387,781	5,612,212
Donor-restricted and Board-designated funds	5,210,377	4,881,029
Total fund balances	10,598,158	10,493,241
Total liabilities and fund balances	$36,960,816	$37,828,280

Exhibit 21.7 Changes in Payer Mix

Type and Source of Revenue	Experience Four Years Ago	Experience Last Year
Percent from SNF operations	38.4%	76.0%
SNF Medicaid revenue	22.0%	35.0%
SNF Medicare revenue	5.0%	8.0%
SNF private pay revenue	73.0%	57.0%

and five are two-bedroom accommodations. Seventy of these units are in the main building, and the other 18 are in cottages, which were added to the campus in the 1950s and early 1960s (see Exhibit 21.2). The main facility, containing residential and assisted living units, is located on two-and-one-quarter acres. The skilled nursing facility is across the street on one-and-one-quarter acres.

The main building of OPRC opened in 1929 as an elegant resort hotel for the rich and famous. The present facade of the main building is considered to be of historic significance, built in the style of an old Spanish courtyard. True to the building's early history and its location by the sea, OPRC still advertises itself as an "elegant, luxurious" facility. Although clean and well-kept, the main lobby actually betrays an old, decaying elegance. In addition, all units are considered small by today's standards, and only the cottages have cooking facilities. None are air conditioned, and none would be considered luxurious by today's standards.

Services and Amenities

A full range of services is offered at OPRC. For those in residential living, the following services are available: three meals per day served in an attractive dining room; housekeeping services twice monthly; scheduled transportation to local shopping, physicians' offices, and cultural events; complete maintenance of interior and exterior facilities; 24-hour emergency services; laundering of bed and bath linens; and personal laundry service for a fee. The retirement community offers a private beach front, a social room for parties and group meetings, lounges, a chapel and chaplaincy services, garden courtyards and walkways, a beauty and barbershop, a library, and a sundry and gift shop. Apartments come in four basic floor plans with wall-to-wall carpeting, drapes, ceiling fans, and cable TV and telephone service prewiring, and have safety rails in the tubs and showers.

Table 21.1 Weekly Campus Occupancy Report (as of April 15, current year)

	Independent Residential Units	Assisted Living Units	Skilled Nursing Units	Total
Ashley Manor	Total Res Avail 137 Total Occupied 103	Total Res Avail 20 Total Occupied 18	Total Res Avail 50 Total Occupied 42	Total Res Avail 207 Total Occupied 163
Ocean Point	Total Res Avail 88 Total Occupied 75	Total Res Avail 13 Total Occupied 10	Total Res Avail 59 Total Occupied 58	Total Res Avail 160 Total Occupied 143
Blue Mountain	Total Res Avail 0 Total Occupied 0	Total Res Avail 62 Total Occupied 53	Total Res Avail 120 Total Occupied 117	Total Res Avail 182 Total Occupied 170
Cedar Grove	Total Res Avail 115 Total Occupied 85	Total Res Avail 48 Total Occupied 39	Total Res Avail 99 Total Occupied 97	Total Res Avail 262 Total Occupied 223
Grand Total Available	340 265	143 120	328 314	811 699

Assisted living units are available for residents who require additional assistance with their daily activities. This includes supervision of medications, help with bathing and dressing as needed, and daily housekeeping service. The OPRC skilled nursing facility compliments the retirement community and is across the street from the main campus. Skilled nursing care is available 24 hours per day, and a physician is on call at all times.

Resident Demographics

A review of OPRC's internal data shows that as of April 1, the average age at admission was 79 (see Exhibit 21.2), a dramatic increase from ten years ago. The average age of residents in the housing units was 85.8 years, and in the skilled nursing facility, 86.3 years. The majority of residents (87 percent) were female and 8 percent were couples. Fifty-five percent lived within a 20 mile radius of OPRC before moving into the facility, and 12 percent lived out of state.

Redevelopment Plans

A task force has been working for nine months to address OPRC's facilities problems. A nationally known consulting firm specializing in the not-for-profit retirement home industry was hired to assess the market area of OPRC and to develop detailed recommendations on unit sizes, amenities and services that would make OPRC financially viable as a retirement community in the future. An architectural firm was engaged both to study what could be done with the existing physical structure at OPRC and to design a complete redevelopment, including demolishing all but the historic facade of the current facilities.

The architectural firm has estimated that making the current facilities comply with seismic codes would cost between $1.2 and $1.4 million. This would still leave the facility with its small uncompetitive units. The organization found that prospective residents for both independent and assisted living often decide to bypass OPRC because of room size and lack of amenities. In the past several years, OPRC has broken through some of the facility walls in order to make larger two-room suites. Although more expensive to rent, these suites were much more in demand than the smaller units. Unfortunately, the building's configuration yields relatively few two-room suites. The monthly fee of a suite is less than the combined monthly fees of two separate units, thereby reducing revenue. For these reasons, supplementing the seismic work on the facility with enlarged units is not a realistic alternative. Ocean Point Retirement Community has also explored alternative uses for its facilities, but financially viable options have not emerged. Some suggested that this be turned into low-income housing for the elderly, but NVH's experience with low-income housing suggests that the occupancy problems would continue.

The consultants' feasibility study suggests that, to survive, OPRC redevelopment should include 150 to 170 upscale congregate apartment units with full kitchens. The need for upscale units is financial. The city of Portwell limits the height of all buildings in the "village" area, where OPRC is located, to two stories. This two-story limit, the relatively small three-and-one-half acre parcel (two-and-one-quarter and one-and-one-quarter) owned by OPRC, the lack of other available land in the vicinity, and the size unit needed to be competitive means relatively few units can be built on the property. Financial proformas prepared by the task force indicate that, for financially viability, the facility must target the well-to-do older population.

They recommended a mix of unit types, with the greatest concentration in one-bedroom with den and two-bedroom apartments. Unit sizes should range from 750 sq. ft. to 1,400 sq. ft. and should have walk-in showers, microwave ovens, balconies or patios with storage, dishwashers, garbage disposals, and laundry appliances. The skilled nursing facility should be completely replaced, and an assisted living component included on the campus. The study also suggested that consideration be given to central spaces accommodating a variety of activities and services (e.g., dining room, library and reading room, outdoor walking and exercise course, and beauty and barber shops).

The redevelopment task force, which includes the consulting firm, the NVH corporate CFO, the administrator of OPRC, a local land-planner, a local financial consultant, and the architects agree that the only feasible alternative is to level the old campus and rebuild. The architects estimate this cannot be done for less than $30 million.

Recent Difficulties

Ocean Point Retirement Community has been experiencing increasingly low occupancy rates. Vacancies over the last ten years have averaged 5.1 percent, and for the last two years over 8 percent. As of April of this year, the overall vacancy rate was 11 percent (the independent residential units were 85 percent occupied, the assisted living 77 percent, and skilled nursing units were at 98 percent occupancy) (see Table 21.1). Admissions over the past ten years have averaged 16.4 new residents per year. The best year was five years ago when 28 new residents were admitted; last year was the worst within this time period, with five new residents. The average for the last two years was only nine admissions per year.

As a result of the low occupancy rate, OPRC has been operating with an increasingly large deficit. The operating deficit last year was $1,006,606 (see Exhibit 21.6). There is no reason to believe that this trend will change, since it appears to be based both on increased competition in South County, and the unappealing size of units and their lack of amenities.

To make matters worse, OPRC has been given a deadline by the city of Portwell to comply with seismic codes. Ocean Point Retirement Community and its parent corporation must decide whether to invest in the old facility, build a new one, or possibly even sell the property.

OPRC's External Environment

Demographics of Primary Market Area

The primary geographic market area was identified by the consulting firm in conjunction with the staff of NVH and OPRC. The primary target market was determined to be persons over age 70 with an annual income in excess of $35,000 apiece. Ocean Point Retirement Community is located in an area with growing numbers of ethnic and racial minorities, primarily Asian and Hispanic (see Table 21.2). Growth within these groups is strongest among the young. In the nonminority groups, the population over age 65 is growing throughout the primary market area. Unlike the national trend, which shows a decline in the population aged 65 to 69 and increases in the older age groups, Portwell's primary market area is experiencing increases in all age groups over 65, with the largest increases in those over the age of 80. Census data from 1990 for the primary market show a pool of 14,853 target households.

The Competition

Ocean Point Retirement Community is faced with more competitors than before, most of which have newer facilities and greater amenities. The total number of residential units, assisted living and Alzheimer units, and skilled nursing beds in the primary market area increased by about 600 percent in the past five years.

Analysis of the competition shows the configurations of retirement communities have increased tremendously and are difficult to categorize. Because OPRC provides multiple levels of care, its competition includes other continuing care retirement communities and rental or condominium retirement communities with services. Some of these provide full apartments with kitchens, offering an independent environment with services, while others are rooms or apartments without cooking facilities. These latter provide three meals per day and are likely to attract a frailer population. Data on licensed and nonlicensed residential care facilities (RCFs)[1] are also included in the analysis.

Table 21.2   Population by Age, Race, and Ethnicity

Demographic data for OPRC primary market are based on the 1990 census and statistical updates for 1992 and 1997.

764,715 people of all ages in primary market area in 1990
Projected population of 961,246 (+26%) for primary market area in 1997
Population of city of Portwell expected to increase from 62,403 to 79,930—1990–1997

Minority Population Numbered 213,862 in 1990

	Percent of Minority Population	Percent of Total Population
Black	13%	4%
Asian	21%	6%
American Indian	3%	1%
Hispanic	63%	18%

Minority Population Estimated at 294,202 for 1997

	Percent of Minority Population	Percent of Total Population	Percent Increase
Black	11%	3%	14%
Asian	20%	6%	38%
American Indian	3%	1%	20%
Hispanic	66%	20%	43%

94,947 people age 65+ in the market area (1990); expected to increase to 125,946 (increase of 33%) by 1997

Age Distribution of the Older Population of the Primary Market Area

Age	1990	1997
65–69	33%	28%
70–74	27%	26%
75–79	20%	21%
80–84	12%	13%
85+	9%	11%

Age Distribution of the Older Population in the City of Portwell

Age	1990	1997
65–69	38%	33%
70–74	28%	28%
75–79	17%	19%
80–84	10%	11%
85+	7%	10%

Continued

Table 21.2   Continued

Households Age 65+

Primary market had 58,064 households age 65+ (headed by someone 65+); 39,646 (68%) were age 70+ and 24,590 (42%) were age 75+ (1990).

Income	Age 65–69	Age 70–74	Age 75+
Under $25,000	6,749	5,585	13,274
$25,000-$35,000	2,930	2,417	3,516
$35,000+	8,790	7,053	7,800

Projected 71,565 households age 65+ in primary market area in 1997, of these 50,801 (71%) will be age 70+ and 35,461 (50%) will be age 75+.

Income	Age 65–69	Age 70–74	Age 75+
Under $25,000	4,652	4,448	13,045
$25,000-$35,000	3,276	3,115	6,314
$35,000+	12,836	7,777	16,102

Seven communities in the primary market area offer both independent living units and nursing home beds. Of these, only one facility (see facility B in Table 21.3) offers continuing care contracts covering unlimited stays in the nursing home for the same monthly fee residents pay in the residential units. The primary market area has 3,717 RCF accommodations in 135 facilities. Most of the licensed capacity (68 percent) is in 14 large facilities, the more than 100 remaining facilities having fewer than ten beds each. There are also a number of facilities for older adults planned for the primary market area, some of which may compete with OPRC, others which may not (see Exhibit 21.8).

Market Survey

A survey was mailed to older households in the market area to gauge the level of interest in moving to a retirement community located at the OPRC site, sponsored by NVH/OPRC. The survey also identified the types of units, services, amenities, and contractual arrangements preferred by potentially interested parties. Returns indicated a high rate of familiarity with OPRC among age and income qualified households. Of all surveys mailed, 7 percent were returned by someone expressing an interest in moving to the facility. Among respondents from the city of Portwell, this figure rose to 12 percent.

Table 21.3 Data on OPRC's Competition

Facilities with both housing and nursing home beds.

Facility	Residential	Assisted	Nursing
A	246	100	59
B	405	21	99
C	57	63	57
D	101	23	59
E	115	—	77
F	98	—	58
OPRC	88	11	59
Total	1,110	218	468

Entry fees at facility B are higher than at OPRC and at facility D, however, facility B is newer and targets a more "upscale" market than the other two facilities.

Facility		Entry Fee	Monthly Fee
B	Studio	$60,480	$950
	One-bedroom	$85,000–118,000	$1,100–1,300
	Two-bedroom	$124,000–190,000	$1,445–2,000
D	Studio	$38,000–42,000	$825–930
	One-bedroom	$47,000–85,000	$955–1,240
	Two-bedroom	$111,000–142,000	$1,500–2,110
OPRC	Studio	$36,000–42,000	$940
	One-bedroom	$66,000–80,000	$1,220
	Two-bedroom	$77,000–95,000	$1,600
A	Studio		None available
	One-bedroom		$2,150
	Two-bedroom		$2,650
C	Studio		None available
	One-bedroom		$1,355–1,589
	Two-bedroom		$1,800
E	Studio		$1,150–1,350
	One-bedroom		$1,625–1,675
	Two-bedroom		$2,275–4,025
F	Studio		$1,375–1,575
	One-bedroom		$1,885
	Two-bedroom		None available

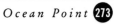

Exhibit 21.8 Planned and Proposed Facilities

....

City of Portwell
Facility P1
Proposed 76-unit development.
14 studio, 56 one-bedroom and 6 two-bedroom apartments.
Permit requires 62 units be affordable housing, 14 can be market rate ($350–$650/month).
Unit sizes range from 267 sq. ft. to 743 sq. ft.
No services planned.
Project must go before City Council in September, current year.

Facility P2
Proposed 170-unit development with a 9,800 sq. ft. community center containing a dining area.
Units: studio 475–522 sq. ft.; one-bedroom 600–745 sq. ft.; two-bedroom 850–1,074 sq. ft.; No units have kitchens.
Common facilities include a pool, reflection pond, tea house (gazebo), walking course and outdoor benches.
Project received approval in March, two years ago. Not acted upon. Permit expired March of current year. To proceed, must go through city approval process again.

Outside of City of Portwell but within Primary Market Area
Facility P3
Failed prior to opening. Currently being converted to 161 units of elderly housing. Units have kitchens. Housing will be affordable and low income. No food service, but under discussion. Future of project unclear.

Facility P4
Single family senior housing. No meals or services provided. Development corporation has filed for Chapter 11, development appears unlikely. Phase I for 175 units approved, Phase II with 350 units has not been approved.

Facility P5
Proposed project for a 71-unit, single family dwelling development. No known progress since receiving approval.

Facility P6
Development at least two years away for this 32-unit single room occupancy project.

Facility P7
In early stages of planning. Ten acres being acquired to develop about 300 units of affordable housing for seniors. Development dependent upon State and Federal tax credits, which will require city support for the project and involvement by a nonprofit entity. Meeting between all concerned parties to be held June 9, current year.

Facility P8
A church is considering building senior housing on property it owns next to the church. No applications have been filed yet.

Continued

Exhibit 21.8   Continued

Facility P9
  240-unit RCFE proposed by development corporation. Approved in December, four
  years ago. Developers trying to sell property but have no strong candidates.

Facility P10
  Expansion of existing facility to include 73 more units of low income housing. Close
  to getting building permits.

Exhibit 21.9   Data on Demand Analysis

In 1992 there were an estimated 18,695 households age 70+ with incomes of $35,000+
in the primary market area. This number is projected to be 23,879 in 1997. Market
penetration rates are based on an analysis of survey returns. Three percent penetration is
considered extremely conservative, 7% is realistic.

Demand Estimates	Age 70–74	Age 75+
Estimated 1994 households	7,615	13,025
Less existing units	−327	−982
Available market pool	7,935	12,043
3% penetration	238	361
5% penetration	397	602
7% penetration	555	843

Consistent with national findings, most respondents showed interest
in larger units with at least one bedroom and a den or two bedrooms.
Most also preferred a full kitchen, although a third of respondents felt
that a kitchen with a microwave and no oven would be adequate. No one
was interested in units without any cooking facilities. Most of OPRC's
current units are extremely small by current standards, and the only units
with cooking facilities are the 18 cottages. The most important factors in
choosing a retirement community were security, cost, quality of services,
and privacy. Surprisingly, beach location was rated "very important" by
only 22 percent of the primary market survey respondents.

Demand Analysis

Based on the estimated number of households for the next year, the data
indicate there will be demand for 599 units at 3 percent penetration rate,
999 units at 5 percent, and 1,398 units at 7 percent penetration for the age
group 70 years and older (see Exhibit 21.9).[2] Of those households with

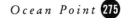

residents 70 years of age and older with income of $35,000 and above that might be interested in moving into a newly developed OPRC, 120 (based on 3 percent penetration) would move in within one to two years. That figure goes to 280 assuming a 7 percent penetration rate. Thus, the near future demand for OPRC is estimated to be between 120 and 280 units.

Conclusion

OPRC and NVH must present the city of Portwell with a plan for OPRC within three months. If nothing is done, the city will condemn the buildings and all residents would have to move elsewhere. Perhaps NVH should help the residents find new facilities, and then sell the valuable ocean front property to a developer. But would this break contractual agreements between NVH and the residents? And what about the initial trust placed in NVH by the congregations of South County that transferred title to NVH free of charge in 1960? They consider OPRC "their" retirement home. If NVH were to sell the property, should the proceeds go toward updating the remaining NVH-owned properties, into development of a new retirement community in inland South County where land is inexpensive, or into expanding services such as home health care?

Redevelopment at the present site will cost at least $30 million. Even if the project is deemed financially feasible and likely to be eventually profitable, should NVH burden itself with such a large debt at a time when the long-term care industry is experiencing financial difficulties? Should management focus a substantial portion of its time and resources on the redevelopment of OPRC while the cutting edge companies in long-term care seem to be expanding their services to include home health care, case management, and outpatient rehabilitation? Of course, a beautifully developed, state-of-the-art oceanside retirement community in Portwell could serve as the flagship for NVH. It could open the door to other profitable developments which could help support NVH's charitable activities. But then again, there are already murmurs of discontent from some of NVH's supporting congregations suggesting that NVH caters to the well-off and does not do enough for the poor elderly. The $30 million development might increase the voices of discontent. What should NVH do with OPRC?

Notes

1. Residential care facilities serve as a bridge between independent living and nursing care. They are sometimes called adult residential facilities, family care, adult foster care, board and care, assisted living, or rest homes.

2. Penetration rates are based on the market's level of interest in retirement housing in Portwell as measured by the survey. Two hundred sixty households with residents 70 years of age and older, of all incomes, expressed interest in moving to OPRC out of 3,776 surveys mailed. This was used as the 7 percent figure. One hundred seven of those interested had incomes of over $35,000, which represents 3 percent of the surveys mailed.

Kidron Bethel Village: Strategic Planning in a Continuing Care Retirement Community

Haris Zafar and James Huxman

Overview

JIM GRABER, president and chief executive officer of Kidron Bethel Retirement Services Incorporated (KBRS) was preparing the agenda for a planning retreat of the Board of Directors. Jim felt that decisions taken at the retreat would be critical to the success of KBRS in the short term, and for continuing success into the twenty-first century.

He had an independent consulting firm prepare an environmental threats and opportunities profile for use by board members during the retreat. He also invited a prominent member of the long-term care professional community in Kansas to serve as facilitator.

Jim wanted to ensure that all board decisions supported the following KBRS mission statement:

> Kidron Bethel Village is a not-for-profit corporation, born from the Mennonite tradition of caring, whose ministry is to provide a full range of retirement services. The Village is an environment which offers security and personal enrichment for those persons 60 years of age and over with opportunities that foster continued growth and development. In serving persons of diverse backgrounds and life situations, Kidron Bethel Village will seek to grow in meeting the changing perceptions of care.

The organization and data are real, but names of individuals are fictitious to assure anonymity.

Evolution of Kidron Bethel Village

With origins in Germany, the deaconess movement among Mennonites in Kansas began as early as 1905. The Bethel Deaconess Home for the Aged was founded in Newton, Kansas, in 1926 by the Western District Conference of the General Conference Mennonite Church. Based on the Mennonite tradition of caring, this facility was integrated with Bethel Deaconess Hospital, founded in 1911. It soon became a model alternative to the county poor farms in the region.

Kidron Incorporated was created in 1979 with a mortgage application to the Department of Housing and Urban Development (HUD) under program section 202. A land option was purchased in North Newton from Bethel College (a Mennonite Church–related four-year, private liberal arts college) for construction, with continuing options for additional parcels for future development. The 1979 application was not accepted by HUD due to the remoteness of the site. However, a second application was made and accepted in 1980. Construction of 55 units of low-income housing for independent living was completed in the summer of 1982, and all apartments were filled within a year. Kidron Bethel Retirement Services Incorporated was formed shortly thereafter.

All of the assets and liabilities, as well as the future operations of the Bethel Deaconess Home for the Aged were received through transfer by the KBRS from the Bethel Deaconess Hospital Association about ten years ago. Responsibility for Kidron Incorporated and any future development on the North Newton Campus was also handed over to KBRS. A new phase of planning for the development of a continuing care retirement community (CCRC), was initiated. A market feasibility study was completed by an outside consulting firm. Based on the assessed needs of the community, construction was completed two years ago on new townhomes, a new intermediate care health care center, and a three-story apartment complex on the North Newton site. Residents of the Bethel Deaconess Home for the Aged were moved to the new facility.

The Current Situation

The Kidron Bethel Village Complex, located in the Newton/North Newton community (population approximately 18,000), consists of the following (see Exhibit 22.1):

1. A three-story condominium building housing 36 apartments, which may be purchased by qualified individuals from KBRS. The condominiums serve a total of 40 people.
2. Kidron Bethel Village duplex townhomes surround the Village on three sides, and may also be purchased by qualified people. Currently,

68 individuals live in 46 duplex townhomes. Upkeep on the duplexes is the responsibility of the Village. Both condominium and townhome owners have access to a two-way voice communication system connected to the health care center. It is monitored 24 hours a day. They also have lifelong access and highest priority to available long-term care beds, if and when total care is needed. By agreement, if the owner later moves to the health care center, or otherwise wishes to sell the unit, KBRS has the first right of refusal to purchase the unit for ninety percent of the owner's base price.

3. Kidron Incorporated, a not-for-profit corporation, provides HUD-subsidized housing for individuals 62 years of age or older who are legally disabled or handicapped. All residents living in Kidron Incorporated must be able to live independently, as nursing care is not included in the offer of housing. Currently, 54 persons are occupying 31 apartments in the main Kidron Incorporated building and six four-plex units across the street from the main building. Maintenance of the grounds is the responsibility of the Village.

4. The Bethel Health Care Center is a 60 bed, private room, intermediate care facility, currently providing 24 hour licensed nursing care to 60 individuals. Short-term care is also offered to individuals requiring temporary care after hospitalization or respite care. Priority is given to individuals over the age of 60 years, but persons who do not meet this requirement are also considered by the board.

5. In addition, KBRS also manages nine off-site apartments that are slated to be phased out, but currently serve nine individuals.

Kidron Bethel Village is currently serving a total of 231 individuals, 68 males and 163 females ranging in age from 46 years to 97 years. While the majority of the residents come from Newton, 38 Kansas counties and 23 other states are represented; one resident is from the Ukraine. The majority of residents are Mennonite, but 14 other religious affiliations are represented.

Kidron Bethel Village offers benefits not often found in other retirement communities. There is an on-site medical clinic, a full-service beauty shop, and a branch bank. The Harvest Table dining facility offers three meals a day. Crafts, woodworking, quilting, monthly social events and day-out trips are offered for all. Health and wellness activities coordinated by a wellness director include general wellness, exercise, and diet programs. There is a fitness room, swimming pool, and a hot tub, and aerobic and aqua aerobic exercise classes are offered regularly.

In summary, Kidron Bethel Village currently provides a full range of services of excellent quality in a caring community within the greater Newton community. There is a continuity of offerings, care, and ease

Exhibit 22.1   Kidron Bethel Village, North Newton, Kansas

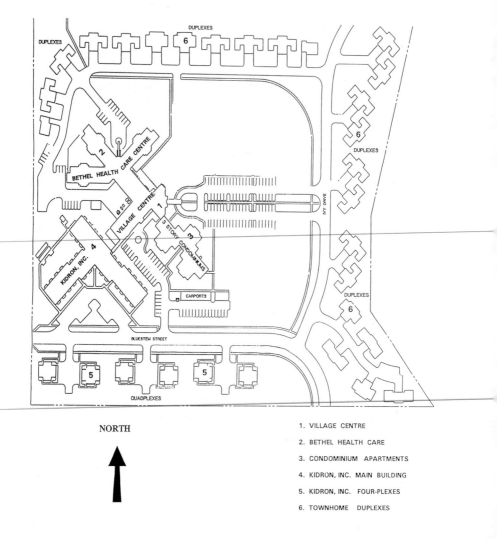

NORTH

1. VILLAGE CENTRE
2. BETHEL HEALTH CARE
3. CONDOMINIUM APARTMENTS
4. KIDRON, INC. MAIN BUILDING
5. KIDRON, INC. FOUR-PLEXES
6. TOWNHOME DUPLEXES

of movement among the facilities as aging changes the needs of the residents.

Current Corporate Organization

Kidron Bethel Retirement Services, Incorporated, is a not-for-profit corporation that operates Kidron Bethel Village. It shares its board of directors with and provides accounting and management services for Kidron Incorporated and Kidron Bethel Condominiums, Inc. (KBC).

Kidron Incorporated pays a management fee to KBRS for accounting and management services, and reimburses KBRS for any specific expenses incurred. Kidron Bethel Condominiums Incorporated is an association for residents of the apartment condominiums and the duplexes. The KBC pays a monthly fee to KBRS for common expenses such as maintenance, utilities, management, and related costs. Figures 22.1 and 22.2 give the current organization structure.

Issues Facing the Board

Jim Graber recently received the results of a needs assessment survey conducted by the same consulting firm which had carried out the original feasibility study. Based on the recommendations of this report, and his own assessment of the situation facing Kidron Bethel Village, he realized that timely decisions would have to be made about the following issues to ensure the continued growth and organizational success of Kidron Bethel Village.

Board of Directors

Jim analyzed the evolution of the board from the original 6 members to its current 13 members. He realized that board member selection was primarily driven by membership in the General Conference Mennonite Church. Of the current 13 members, all but three are Mennonite, and there are only three women. The goal of board member selection remains to ensure community and financial support while retaining ties with the four General Conference Mennonite Churches in the Newton community.

The membership of the current board is strongly representative of the populations being served by the Village. They are as follows:

1. Church-affiliated members (four)
2. Contributors, those individuals who have contributed at least $100 to the Village (three)
3. Individuals selected at large from the Newton Community (three)
4. Residents, from members of the condominium association (three).

Six members of the current board have teaching backgrounds at the college level; three of these six individuals are in Seminary education. There are two members who are in senior positions in finance at local businesses. The rest of the board consists of a retired pastor, a retired owner of a hardware store, a retired farmer, one person in industrial sales, and one individual in an editorial position with the Mennonite General Conference.

Figure 22.1 Kidron Bethel Retirement Services, Inc., Organization Chart

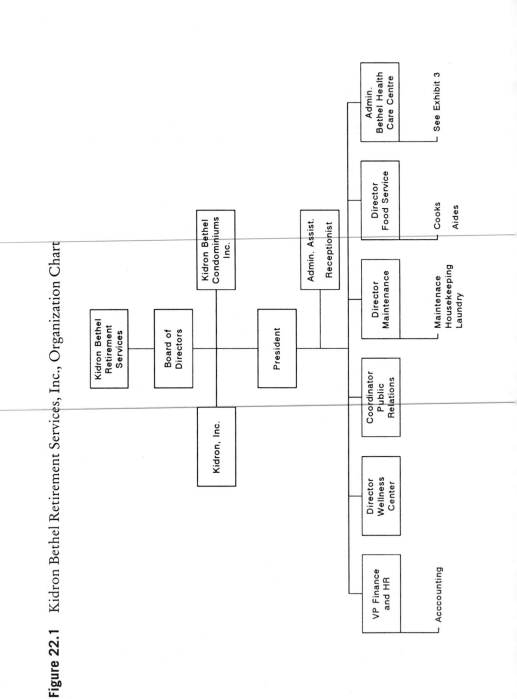

Figure 22.2 Bethel Health Care Centre Organization Chart

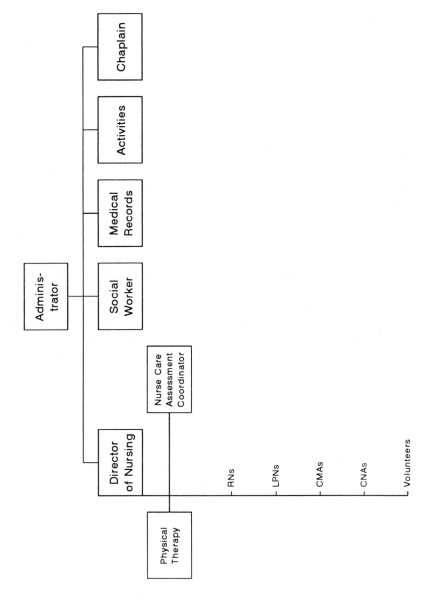

Jim worked very closely with the nominating committee of the board for the last two years to ensure that the members selected to serve the three-year terms on the board had a broad range of expertise. Jim felt that in order to meet the challenges being posed by health care reform and future expansion issues faced by the organization, the board must be represented in the areas of finance, health care delivery, construction, and legislative process. He was not sure if more diversity was needed, or if the existing board composition of affiliations and expertise was adequate.

Finance

The major source of financial support for Kidron Bethel has been the Western District Conference of the General Conference Mennonite Church. Financial support from the regional conference has continually declined, and currently the four local Mennonite Churches are the primary contributors. This decline in church support is understandable, since Mennonite communities have built local nursing homes and provide financial support to them.

It can be clearly seen from financial statements that in the last few years there have been substantial losses (see the Comparative Balance Sheets and Comparative Statements of Revenue and Expenses of KBRS for the last four years in Table 22.1 and Table 22.2).

In part, these large losses can be attributed to writing off the assets of the Bethel Deaconess Home for the Aged. This facility had to be demolished, since attempts to sell it were unsuccessful, however, KBRS still retains the land. Substantial financial reserves were also used in the building of the North Newton Campus.

Another financial issue which must be carefully dealt with is that of bidding for Medicaid beds, required since Kansas is a participant in a new case-mix project. The 60-bed Bethel Health Care Center definitely will feel the impact. Kansas, Michigan, Maine, and South Dakota are the four states participating in the Medicaid portion of the case-mix project. Texas and New York, in addition to the previous four states, are participating in the Medicare portion of the project. This reimbursement methodology is supposed to be fully phased in by July of the current year in Kansas.

There are currently four cost centers, including the administrative cost center, the health care cost center, the plant and operating cost center, and the room and board cost center. In order to determine the Medicaid payment methodology to the nursing facilities, Medicaid establishes caps in each of the four cost centers. In the administrative cost center, the cap is set at the 75th percentile of all nursing facilities. This cap is calculated by taking the administrative cost of all nursing facilities and eliminating

Table 22.1 Comparative Balance Sheets

	Last Year	2 Years Ago	3 Years Ago	4 Years Ago
Assets				
Current assets				
Cash and equivalents	$ 305,806	$ 261,773	$ 521,666	$ 351,523
Certificates of deposit	124,026	—	—	—
Assets whose use is limited and are required for current liabilities (Note 1)	170,372	168,171	98,171	98,171
Accounts receivable, residents	71,447	71,937	68,755	65,242
Due from Kidron, Inc.	2,365	9,321	—	4,163
Due from Kidron Bethel Condominiums, Inc.	25,620	—	—	—
Note receivable	—	109,243	—	—
Housing construction (Note 2)				
Contracts receivable	39,613	85,947	897,515	1,086,131
Living units	111,188	472,341	—	—
Construction costs	—	—	495,552	1,044,466
Prepaid expenses and other	24,563	17,917	11,820	11,947
Total current assets	$ 875,000	1,196,650	2,093,479	2,661,643
Assets whose use is limited (Note 1)	86,092	88,489	992,986	2,654,331
Property assets, less accumulated depreciation (Note 3)	3,559,523	3,719,420	2,883,880	1,223,735
Other assets	124,617	156,681	262,613	269,289
Total	$4,645,232	$5,161,240	$6,232,958	$6,808,998

Continued

Table 22.1 Continued

	Last Year	2 Years Ago	3 Years Ago	4 Years Ago
Liabilities and Fund Balances				
Current liabilities				
Current portion of long-term debt	$ 118,738	$ 383,311	$ 37,085	$ 34,445
Accounts payable	85,982	130,132	157,203	228,991
Accrued payroll	78,303	69,159	61,013	48,719
Accrued interest payable	95,372	98,171	98,171	98,171
Other accrued liabilities	50,995	13,283	13,563	12,844
Deferred revenue—				
Housing contracts (Note 2)	—	80,000	966,168	1,558,013
Insurance proceeds and other	18,652	50,598	39,454	—
Due to Kidron Bethel Condominiums, Inc.	54,986	—	—	—
Total current liabilities	503,028	824,654	1,372,657	1,981,183
Annuities payable (Note 4)	12,494	13,321	14,385	17,134
Estimated unemployment costs (Note 5)	69,296	51,806	34,589	20,601
Long-term debt (Note 6)	2,949,498	3,081,210	3,178,574	3,215,659
Total liabilities	3,534,316	3,970,991	4,600,205	5,234,577

Fund balances				
General	849,827	976,869	1,475,170	1,463,793
Restricted	261,089	213,380	157,583	110,628
Total fund balances	1,110,916	1,190,249	1,632,753	1,574,421
Total	$4,645,232	$5,161,240	$6,232,958	$6,808,998

NOTES

1. *Assets whose use is limited:* The city of Newton issued $3,000,000 of 20-year Healthcare Facilities Revenue Bonds five years ago for the purpose of constructing and equipping certain facilities to be leased to KBRS and which may be purchased by KBRS for a nominal amount at the end of the lease term. A designated trustee received the bond issue proceeds, receives the lease payments from KBRS, and disburses the monies in accordance with a trust indenture agreement.

2. *Housing construction:* KBRS records the sale of a unit at the later of the closing of the sale or the completion of construction of a unit. Living units not sold are recorded at their construction cost.

3. *Property, plant, and equipment:* Property, plant, and equipment are recorded at cost or at net book value if transferred from a related organization. Depreciation is provided on the straight-line method utilizing useful lives ranging from 5 to 40 years.

4. *Annuities payable:* Annuities payable represent the present value of the interest payments on the principal of annuity contracts with individuals until death of the annuitant at which time the principal becomes a donation to KBRS as specified by the annuitant.

5. *Estimated unemployment costs:* KBRS is self-insured for its unemployment insurance and pays unemployment benefits to the State of Kansas for claims received each quarter. KBRS records as a liability an amount that approximates the unemployment insurance that would have been due the State of Kansas if KBRS were a participating employer. Payments for benefits are charged against liability.

6. *Long-term debt:* This consists of the following; note payable to a local commercial lender collateralized by apartment building, special assessment for KBRS' share of improvements for streets, sewer, and water payable to the City of North Newton, capital lease obligation City of North Newton, Healthcare facilities revenue bonds collateralized by leased facilities and equipment, line of credit interest payments with a local bank secured by a real estate mortgage.

Table 22.2 Comparative Statements of Revenue and Expenses

	Last Year	2 Years Ago	3 Years Ago	4 Years Ago
Operating Revenue				
Resident service revenue, net of provision for bad debts and contractual allowances of $66,009 ($111,289; 127,649; 105,260 for previous years)	$1,569,552	$1,318,098	$1,338,147	$1,221,824
Entrance fees	38,097	35,337	—	—
Kidron Bethel Condominiums, Inc., net of direct expenses	194,977	150,792	—	—
Other	110,696	82,853	58,441	35,016
Total operating revenue	$1,913,322	1,587,080	1,396,588	1,256,840
Operating Expenses				
Nursing service	757,275	701,808	592,899	549,153
Dietary	367,731	350,448	241,673	242,413
General services	409,664	372,872	305,042	258,861
Administrative services	289,210	324,979	356,079	286,228
Depreciation and amortization	194,201	139,946	66,365	69,846
Interest	253,942	153,307	21,732	17,838
Total operating expenses	2,272,023	2,043,360	1,583,790	1,424,339
Loss from operations	(358,701)	(456,280)	(187,202)	(167,499)

Non-operating Revenue (Expenses)

Investment income				
Farm & rental properties, net	5,849	25,028	27,553	17,565
Interest	20,826	33,654	26,592	33,569
Gain, investment property sales	16,122	44,493	—	—
Contributions	61,505	76,960	32,294	7,274
Entrance Fees				
Kidron Bethel Condominiums, Inc., net of direct expenses	—	—	64,018	15,429
Income from residence sales	127,357	182,556	10,685	63,230
Loss on discontinued premises (Note 1)	—	(404,712)	—	—
Non-operating revenue, net	231,659	(42,012)	198,579	236,094
Excess (deficit) of revenue over expenses	($ 127,042)	($498,301)	$ 11,377	$ 68,595

NOTE

1. *Loss on discontinued premises*: KBRS demolished the Bethel Deaconess Home for the Aged, after unsuccessful attempts to sell. Land is still retained by KBRS.

those facilities which have costs higher than the 75th percentile. The health care cost center cap is set at the 90th percentile, the room and board cost center is set at the 90th percentile, and the plant and operating cost center is set at the 85th percentile.

Case-mix reimbursement will radically change this formula. The new reimbursement methodology will establish an administrative cap at the 55th percentile, a health care cost center cap at the 60th percentile, a plant and operating cost center cap at the 55th percentile, and room and board cost center cap at the 60th percentile.

Based upon level of care, each facility will have a case-mix index. The case-mix index is a facility average index that is derived from MDS Plus assessment data. The state average is 1.00. If a facility's index is higher than 1.00, then the facility's resident care needs are higher than average. Each facility is reimbursed according to the level of care being given to its residents. Kidron Bethel has a case-mix index of less than 1.00 and would stand to loose an excess of fifty thousand dollars per year under the new system.

This type of revenue reduction has significant implications for future staffing, rate increases in the facility, and continued participation in the Medicaid program. Further, Kidron Bethel is also facing implications of 50/50 Medicaid/self-pay Mix, rather than the 35/65 mix internally projected for initial planning purposes.

The financial challenge had taken on such magnitude and importance that Jim, with the Board's approval, just hired a vice president of Finance and Human Resources. Jim knew that something had to be done soon to make the financial statements look better, since community confidence in management might decline if nothing were changed.

Competition

Kidron Bethel Village is one of four large CCRCs in the city of Newton. The other three are Presbyterian Manor, with 60 intermediate care beds and 47 independent living units; Kansas Christian Home with 115 intermediate care beds and 26 independent living units, and Friendly Acres (Methodist) with 144 intermediate care beds; 46 licensed personal care beds, and 90 independent living units.

KBRS board members must decide if they should build apartments, duplexes, or assisted living units. The land for new construction is available. The demand for independent living units with an option for long-term care was evident to Jim from the waiting list of over 200 individuals who had already paid one thousand dollars each as a deposit.

New Program Development

With health care reform suggesting potentially increased funding for home and community-based services, should KBRS forego construction and focus on program development—specifically home health services? Currently, two of the local CCRCs have their own home health agencies, and the city of Newton also has a community home health service.

When the Kidron Bethel Village Complex was built, the board decided to offer independent living and a total care continuum. The residents, as a community, refused to support accepting assistive services at that time. The board, thus, decided not to pursue the assisted living service option. Presently, Kidron Bethel Village is the only CCRC in the community not licensed for personal care and assisted living, and is at a severe disadvantage as a result.

Based on the needs assessment report, Jim felt that residents were more accepting of the reality of "aging in place," and 95 percent who responded to a survey thought that the available space should be used for building assisted care units. Jim also felt a strong support for assisted living services being provided by KBRS in the independent living units.

Jim put these four issues on the agenda for the upcoming retreat and felt confident that the meeting would result in solutions to these issues. He felt there would be a renewed focus on Kidron Bethel Village to make it an even more vibrant and thriving total care community in the face of the challenges and opportunities of the future.

Angel Crest Manor: For Love or Money?

Raymond Alan Mattes and Kathleen H. Wilber

WESLEY JOHNSON, chief operating officer of Gabriel Care Homes, Inc. (GCH), slouched in his chair, deep in thought. His eyes solemnly surveyed the small needlepoint plaque hanging on the wall opposite his desk. It had been given to him by a 96-year-old resident shortly after he began working for the corporation. Over the years, its message, "Care—In all Ways for all Time" had become his personal motto. This message also reflects the organization's Mission Statement (Exhibit 23.1). Today was the annual board meeting, and a decision was expected concerning the fate of the corporation's oldest retirement facility, Angel Crest Manor (ACM).

The preceding months had been filled with uncertainty and turmoil. The most recent disaster was simply another crisis in a series of events that had challenged the facility in recent years. ACM was the corporation's birthplace. Service by the Sisters of St. Mary of the Angels to those in need of extended care began on that small campus in the heart of the city over 90 years ago. Today's meeting would determine whether or not service would continue at ACM. Having spent over two years examining corporate records, financial statements, and reimbursement projections; conducting feasibility studies; and reviewing demographic reports, Wesley Johnson wrestled with the reality of an organization struggling to stay true to its original mission in a rapidly changing environment.

Fictitious names of both the organization and individuals are used to assure anonymity. Facts and issues were modified to enhance teaching value.

Note: The authors wish to thank Sandy Reynolds for assistance with the graphics.

Exhibit 23.1 Mission and Philosophy Statement of Gabriel Care Homes, Inc.

At Gabriel Care Homes, Inc., we believe we have a duty to respond to Gospel values of serving our neighbor in justice, charity and good-will; therefore, in the spirit of our foundress, any elderly individual who approaches us for care, regardless of race, creed, nationality, sex, handicap, or economic status is entitled to share the fruits of our ministry in comfortable supportive surroundings. We pledge to provide elderly residents with CARE—IN ALL WAYS FOR ALL TIME.

Background

ACM began in 1902 as Angel Crest Home for Aged and Infirm Women. Founded by the Sisters of St. Mary of the Angels, its first administrator, Sister Mary Gabriel, established its mission as the provision of compassionate care and shelter to poor, aged, and infirm women. The mission was revised to broaden the definition of those in need. ACM was incorporated as Gabriel Care Homes, Inc., in 1950. One of the sisters was named president of the new corporation, whose Board of Directors was made up of community leaders.

Over the years new buildings were constructed with philanthropic gifts from grateful families and a supportive community. As the number of sisters in the community declined, lay persons became more predominant in the staffing of ACM. In 1965, the sisters turned over organizational management to the laity, while retaining sponsorship and some decision-making authority.

ACM was the first of six facilities owned and operated by Gabriel Care Homes, Inc. GCH's goal is to provide senior adults comfortable surroundings, supportive services, and maintained independence. Until 1950, the corporation supported residential care through bequests, the family estate of one of the sisters, and fundraising proceeds. It enjoyed a reputation for the high quality of its residential care. After incorporation, life-care contracts were introduced to residents at ACM through which residents paid an entry fee to ensure care during their lifetime. Currently, all accommodations are available to residents through a fee-for-service plan.

In the late 1960s, the corporation acquired retirement facilities in California, Nevada, and Arizona, but rapid growth and poor actuarial projections yielded financial difficulty during the 1970s. This nearly forced the corporation to file for bankruptcy, and resulted in several lawsuits by residents and major corporate restructuring. A financial settlement forced the corporation to sell its out-of-state facilities, take several loans to honor existing life-care contracts, and as part of the restructuring, accept Ian Newman as the first lay president, replacing Sister Mary Elizabeth. Newman had extensive experience in the for-profit nursing home sector and the hotel and hospitality industries. He had a reputation for his belief that form follows funding, attention to the bottom line, and his ability to salvage floundering enterprises. The Sisters of St. Mary of the Angels retained 5 of 13 votes on the restructured board of directors, hoping to preserve the mission and philosophy of the organization.

By 1980, life-care contract residents in all six facilities were affected by the corporation's financial difficulties, but ACM residents were affected the most, due to their higher average age (6.8 years) and greater number of impairments in activities of daily living (which had increased by 30 percent). The corporation agreed to charge each life-contract resident a reduced monthly rate for continual care, in essence providing a loan to the corporation until full financial restructuring could occur. Residents (or heirs) would be repaid these additional funds, with interest, upon withdrawal from the facility or death. The corporation's financial position improved, and it took steps to obtain a competitive edge in a difficult market.

The five facilities acquired during the 1960s and 1970s primarily served well-to-do residents. ACM differed from the other facilities. Its institutional "look" reflected a religious mission of altruism, love, compassion, and service to elders, with financial need as the sole determinant of admission. Over the years, the corporation had expanded its service base from exclusively low-income individuals to include all older adults.

During the 1980s, concern for the overall well-being of each resident as an essential mission appeared to be giving way to a push for market share and strategic expansion. Emphasis shifted from philanthropic service to running the company like a business. A strategic plan was developed, a capital campaign launched, and assets directed toward cosmetic remodeling of the facility. Marketing themes depicted "a home for loved ones in an elegant environment." Sections of the facility began to resemble a hotel instead of a long-term care community. While some staff appeared to delight in the improvements, the morale of other long-term employees suffered, with some leaving in frustration over the drastic changes. One nurse commented that after the restructuring, "ACM became just another bureaucratic, greedy, and uncaring place." Other employees felt the emphasis placed on remodeling was a refreshing change from the era when funds went primarily for the care of needy

Figure 23.1 Angel Crest Manor

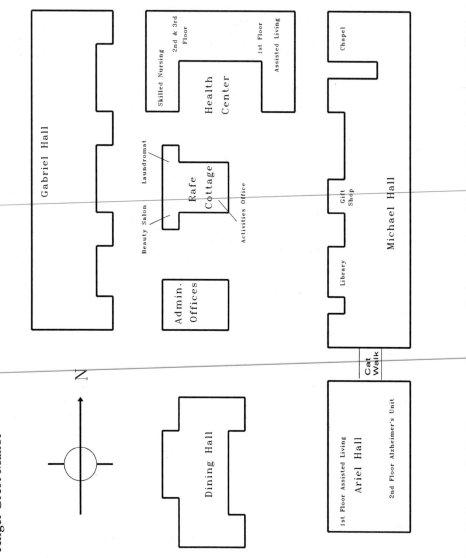

residents. One remarked, "the new changes make coming to work a nice experience, and the residents and their families love it."

The Campus

Angel Crest Manor evolved as the residents' needs changed. The original, large two-story residence housing 20 women was expanded, adding small cottages around the central building. Larger units were added, each designed for specific needs of the time, with little consideration given to future needs of the facility or residents, which resulted in a dysfunctional campus.

Physically, ACM is a self-enclosed campus housing independent and assisted living, and a skilled nursing facility. Most of the 200 residents live in the independent living section. Their average age is 84 and most are single or widowed with no children. Within the system, ACM has the highest occupancy rate, proportion of residents on Supplemental Security Income (SSI) in independent and assisted living, and proportion on Medicaid in the skilled nursing facility. It has always maintained a high profile in the community, whose organizations have made numerous referrals over the years.

ACM's resident population has become increasingly ethnically and socioeconomically diverse. While its marketing efforts center on its surrounding community, the five other corporate facilities engage in nationwide marketing strategies geared toward attracting private pay residents from the east coast to experience "gracious retirement living in a caring and compassionate environment" in the sun belt.

The three-story skilled nursing unit is in the Health Center (see Figure 23.1). The skilled nursing administrator's office, medical records, business office, and the facility's clinic are located on the first floor. The clinic is open daily until 3 p.m., serving both independent and assisted living residents. The clinic is staffed by an LPN and two nursing assistants. Clinic staff are the first to respond with medical attention to an emergency or accident. Some assisted living resident rooms are also located on this floor. The second and third floors contain 51 skilled beds.

Ariel Hall, across the campus from the nursing unit, is a two-story structure that is home to residents needing assistance with activities of daily living or suffering from dementia-related disorders. Its second floor is designated as the Alzheimer's Unit, the first of its kind in the area. Second floor residents must either climb the stairs or use an elevator in the main building, and walk across a catwalk to their rooms.

The main building, Michael Hall, is a four-story residential apartment building housing a council room, a gift shop, a library, and a central

Figure 23.2 Gabriel Care Homes, Inc.
Organization Chart

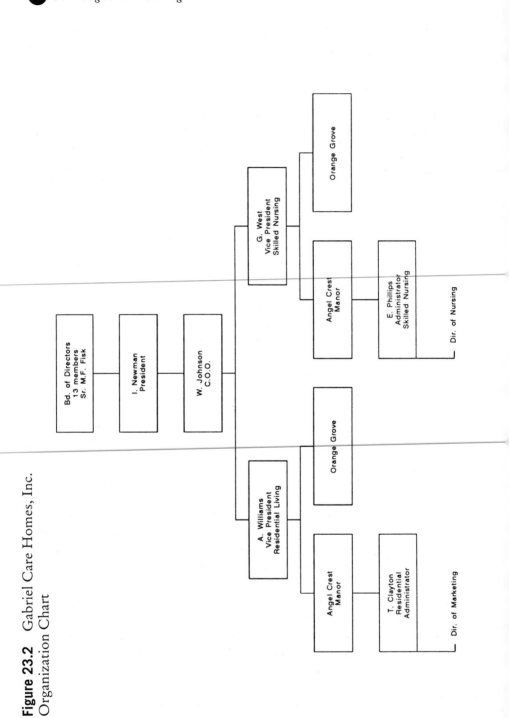

lounge, that connects to the stately chapel. Other buildings on the campus include Gabriel Hall, a six-story independent residential apartment building; the dining hall; Rafe Cottage, which houses the activities department, exercise room, residential laundry facilities, and beauty salon; and Administration Cottage, which houses the administrator's office, as well as the marketing, business, accounting, and personnel offices.

As an inner-city retirement community, ACM has seen many changes. The surrounding neighborhood, once the hub of social life for the more affluent members of the area, is now home to a large number of recent immigrants from Korea, Russia, Armenia, Mexico, and Central America. Check-cashing stores and pawn shops are intermingled with businesses catering to the new immigrant's needs. Billboards, street signs, and shop windows bear advertisements in several languages. Many of the facility's employees are drawn from the local community and from other low-income neighborhoods accessible by bus.

The community has seen a dramatic increase in the number of residents requiring personal care assistance, creating unexpected conflict within the facility. Some of the independent residents resent the admission of new frail residents, viewing their dependence as a reflection of the facility's overall decline. As the pool of private pay residents decreased, the marketing staff recruited residents from the surrounding neighborhood, many of whom are on SSI.

A waiting list exists for assisted living. Increasingly, residents are admitted to independent living only to be evaluated several months later as incapable of functioning alone. In many cases, the resident remains in independent living and receives personal care services until a room is available in the assisted living section. Waiting time ranges from several months to a year.

Organizational Structure

Angel Crest Manor is a division within GCH, Inc. Reporting to the board and president is the chief operating officer, Wesley Johnson (see Figure 23.2). The vice president of residential living, Alice Williams, oversees all residential and assisted living units of the six Gabriel Care Homes. The vice president of skilled nursing, George West, oversees the corporation's three nursing facilities.

Within ACM, the residential facility and skilled nursing facility have separate co-equal administrators supervised by their respective corporate officers. The administrator of the residential section, Thomas Clayton, oversees independent living, assisted living, pastoral care, maintenance, the clinic, housekeeping, dining services, the business and accounting office, the personnel office, marketing, and activities.

Eric Phillips oversees nursing services and medical records specifically for the skilled nursing center. Phillips is the third administrator of the skilled nursing facility in the past two years. There are no assistant administrators. The director of marketing reports to the residential administrator; the director of nursing reports to the skilled nursing administrator.

Changing Environment

Several years ago, ACM found itself in the middle of urban rioting. Residents stood by their windows and watched as shops were looted and buildings burned only a block away. Several tense days brought fear and uncertainty. Given the visible presence of street gangs and frequent sounds of gun shots, police sirens, and surveillance helicopters that are now a part of everyday life, many residents gave up outside activities, preferring to remain within the safe confines of the campus.

The Earthquake

Two months ago a major earthquake jolted residents of ACM awake before dawn, damaging power lines, and cutting electricity to all but the skilled nursing facility. The uncertainty of the event, the early hour at which it occurred, lack of emergency drills, and the inability to see in the darkened buildings prevented many staff members from performing their duties. A few residents wandered the halls, others nervously chatted while waiting for instructions. Most, out of fear, did not venture out of their apartments.

Shortly after the main shock, staff set about the task of examining the campus and the condition of the residents. Many windows in the skilled nursing facility and the large solarium window in Gabriel Hall were shattered. Structural damage was evident in the stairwell leading to the third floor of the skilled nursing unit, as were cracks throughout the facility. Shattered windows, many in rooms occupied by residents, were left unattended until late the following afternoon.

Neither administrator could reach the facility on the day of the earthquake. Eric Phillips arrived two days after the quake to meet with corporate representatives. Wesley Johnson, accompanied by Alice Williams, toured the facility on the day of the earthquake to assess damage.

The most severe damage occurred in Michael Hall where the third and fourth floors connect to the chapel. Apartments on both floors were damaged. The apartment of one resident, who had been admitted to a rehabilitation hospital before the earthquake, revealed a vast amount of structural damage. Parts of a supportive pillar had fallen onto his bed. Large wooden bookcases and shelves lay in pieces on the floor. An eight-inch crack in the solid concrete wall spread from the fourth to the third floors. Shifting caused the floor to buckle in several areas. Residents living in damaged areas were moved to vacant apartments throughout the facility. Two days after the earthquake, the last resident with a damaged apartment was moved to safer quarters.

The hours immediately following the earthquake were filled with confusion. News reports warned of contaminated water, continued loss of electricity, and interrupted phone service. Residents were uncertain how to react to the often conflicting directives in the news reports. Conflicts and angry outbursts were common. Residents lashed out at employees, especially those with whom they had the most contact, such as housekeepers and maintenance personnel. Four days later, counselors were brought in to conduct seminars, in English, to assist employees in confronting any fears or anxieties they might have had because of the earthquake.

A week after the earthquake, corporate engineers surveyed the buildings of ACM. Thomas Clayton accompanied them on his first day back at the facility. Yellow strips indicating "caution" cordoned off the area directly in front of the chapel where the most serious damage had occurred. The remaining buildings were structurally sound. New windows were ordered for the skilled nursing facility and the solarium. Fortunately, the facility had adequate earthquake insurance to cover the preliminary damage estimate of $1.7 million.

Over the next few weeks, life slowly returned to a normal pace at ACM as the facility prepared for the annual board of directors meeting. Staff returned to normal work schedules, activities and resident outings resumed, but signs of strain and discontent persisted. Six private pay residents moved to other facilities. The families of several others threatened to remove their loved ones if changes to the facility's approach to emergencies and assurance of its safety and repair were not adequately addressed. At the monthly resident council meeting, the administrator suggested that, due to the poor response during the earthquake, more extensive training would be required of floor captains. Two residents on the council resigned in protest over the lack of proper guidelines and directives in disaster situations, charging that economic factors were the reason so few staff members had been on duty during the night shift when the earthquake had struck.

Annual Board Meeting

ACM's future was given priority on this year's board agenda. Wesley Johnson, with results of his study in hand, could only guess what would happen at the meeting. Data indicated that, while ACM maintained an occupancy rate of 98 percent, endowment funds were increasingly needed to offset annual operating deficits. ACM's reimbursement rates were significantly below those of the other five facilities that are part of Gabriel Care Homes, Inc. The feasibility study focused on remodeling floors in Michael and Gabriel Halls currently containing one- and two-bedroom apartments into studio apartments, in anticipation of increasing numbers of low-income residents.

Several options faced the board of directors. ACM could be sold, thereby alleviating any future problems for Gabriel Care Homes, Inc. This option was supported by some board members with a business interest, but not favored by the sisters. Another option was to restore the facility with earthquake insurance funds, hoping the future would yield community development projects to enhance the surrounding neighborhoods.

The third option, promoted by Sister Mary Francis Fisk, the chairperson of the board, was that the board champion the original ACM mission by concentrating its resources on the community and low-income individuals. She argued repeatedly that the corporation had weathered its financial crisis in the late 1970s mistakenly by drifting away from its original mission. She was not about to let this happen again, and stated that, "it is unconscionable to deny our elders the care they need simply because they lack the means to pay for it."

Sister Mary Francis saw the reputation of the corporation and her entire order as being at stake in this issue. She proposed using the earthquake insurance money to begin to make modifications in the physical plant, while continuing to subsidize ACM until it was able to become more self-sufficient. She believed innovative programming and sound, no-frills management would pay off. She advocated expansion of the assisted living area for low-income individuals and those suffering from Alzheimer's-related disorders to serve the unmet needs of the immediate neighborhood. She also proposed expanding the services offered by the clinic to the surrounding community and the development of a state-of-the-art adult day care program. The clinic could be utilized by individuals in the neighborhood who were in need of in-home care. Day care would provide respite for local caregivers, as well as serve older persons who lived alone. A recent needs assessment contracted by the Area Agency on Aging had indicated strong need for these services.

Sister Mary Francis suggested the board consider several strategies to increase revenue at the facility, including investigating the development of a contract with a local hospital to provide subacute care, aggressive fundraising to increase the facility's endowment, and a state grant to support day care. According to Sister Mary Francis, the core ACM mission is on-target, but must be adapted to meet changing long-term care needs.

The meeting is scheduled to begin in a few minutes in the council room of ACM. Pausing in front of Michael Hall, Wesley Johnson gazes at the barricaded chapel area, where the structural damage is still very apparent, and contemplates the irony of the situation. Would this most recent crisis mean opportunity or catastrophe for the original facility, its residents, and staff?

List of Contributors

William E. Aaronson, Ph.D.
Department of Health
  Administration
Temple University
Philadelphia, PA

James E. Allen, Ph.D.
Department of Health Policy and
  Administration
University of North Carolina
Chapel Hill, NC

Lois Bluhm, R.N., M.H.A.
Corporate Nursing Coordinator
Certified Gerontological Nurse
  (ANA)
Health Care Capital, Inc.
Shreveport, LA

Keith Boles, Ph.D.
Associate Professor
Program in Health Services
  Management
University of Missouri—
  Columbia

Gerald N. Cohn
Executive Vice President
Wesner Heritage Village
Columbus, OH

Miriam Cotler, Ph.D.
Professor
Health Administration Program
Department of Health Science
California State University,
  Northridge

Catherine Crowley
Clinical Manager
Subacute/Skilled Nursing Facility
Holy Cross Medical Center
Mission Hills, CA

Robert H. Daugherty
Consultant
Louisville, KY

Diane K. Duin, M.H.A.
Instructor
Department of Health Services
  Administration
University of South Dakota
Vermillion, SD

Neil Dworkin, Ph.D.
Associate Director
United Hebrew Geriatric Center
New Rochelle, NY

Jan M. Fritz, Ph.D., C.C.S.
Associate Professor
College of Design, Architecture,
   Art, and Planning
School of Planning
University of Cincinnati
Cincinnati, OH

Margaret Hastings, Ph.D.
Policy and Management Institute
Kenilworth, IL

Marc D. Hiller, Dr.P.H.
Associate Professor and
Director of Undergraduate Studies
Department of Health
   Management and Policy
University of New Hampshire
Durham, NH

James Huxman
President
Kidron Bethel Village
Wichita, KS

Donna Lind Infeld, Ph.D.
Professor
Department of Health Services
   Management and Policy
The George Washington
   University
Washington, DC

James A. Irvin, Ph.D.
Director, Center for Study of
   Aging
Associate Professor
Program in Health Services
   Management
University of Missouri—
   Columbia
Columbia, MO

Bonnie S. Kantor, Sc.D.
Director, Office of Geriatrics and
   Gerontology
College of Medicine
Ohio State University
Columbus, OH

Jeffrey A. Kramer, Ph.D.
Director and Assistant Professor
Center for Health Systems
   Management
University of Connecticut
Storrs, CT

John R. Kress, M.H.A.
Director of Long-Term Care and
   Aging
Association of University
   Programs in Health
   Administration
Arlington, VA

Sue Lehrman
Union College
Graduate Management Institute
Schnectady, NY

James B. Lewis, Sc.D.
Assistant Professor
Health Management and Policy
University of New Hampshire
Durham, NH

Raymond Alan Mattes, B.A.
Research Assistant
Andrus Gerontology Center
University of Southern California
Los Angeles, CA

Patricia McCormack, R.N.,
   M.S.N.
Vice President of Nursing
United Hebrew Geriatric Center
New Rochelle, NY

Robert C. Myrtle, D.P.A.
Professor
Health Services Administration
   Program
University of Southern California
Los Angeles, CA

Alice L. O'Neill, Ed.D., N.H.A.
Department of Human
   Resources
University of Scranton
Scranton, PA

Arnold M. Possick, M.H.A.,
   M.S.G.
Director, Senior Services
Greater Valley Medical Group
Mission Hills, CA

Janet Reagan, Ph.D.
Professor
Department of Health Science
Califorina State University—
   Northridge
Northridge, CA

William T. Reddick, Ph.D.
Assistant Professor
Department of Health Services
   Administration
University of South Dakota
Vermillion, SD

Kent V. Rondeau
Assistant Professor
Faculty of Health Professions
School of Health Services
   Administration
Dalhousie University
Halifax, Nova Scotia, Canada

Pamela P. Sawyer, M.H.A.
Regional Director
Special Care
Woburn, MA

Diane P. S. Shipe, M.H.A., Ph.D.
Assistant Professor
Department of Health Sciences
James Madison University
Harrisonburg, VA

Henry W. Smorynski, Ph.D.
Professor, Political Science
Vice President for Academic
   Affairs
Lewis University
Romeoville, IL

William F. Sturtevant
Administrator
Rockingham County Nursing
   Home
Brentwood, NH

Donna D. VanIwaarden, Ph.D.
Assistant Professor
Health Administration
   Coordinator
Grand Valley State University
Grand Rapids, MI

Kathleen H. Wilber, Ph.D.
Assistant Professor of
  Gerontology and Public
  Policy
Leonard Davis School of
  Gerontology
University of Southern California
Los Angeles, CA

Haris Zafar, M.B.A., Ph.D.
President
Audiology and Hearing Aid
  Services, Inc.
Wichita, KS

Jacqueline S. Zinn, Ph.D.
Assistant Professor
Department of Health
  Administration
Temple University
Philadelphia, PA

About the Editors

Donna Lind Infeld, Ph.D., is Professor of Health Services Management and Policy and of Health Care Sciences, specializing in Long-Term Care Administration, at The George Washington University, where she was recently Senior Associate Dean of the School of Business and Public Management. She has been at the George Washington University since completing her Ph.D. in Social Welfare at the Heller School at Brandeis University in 1978. In addition to long-term care administration courses, she teaches in the areas of Program Evaluation and Research Methods, Health Information Systems, Human Behavior and Human Resources. Dr. Infeld is Editor of *The Hospice Journal* and treasurer of the Gerontological Society of America (GSA). She was previously chair of the GSA Social Research, Planning and Practice Section and a member of the District of Columbia Board of Examiners for Nursing Home Administrators. She also chaired the AUPHA Long-Term Care Administration Education Project advisory committees. She has coedited two books: *Cases in Long-Term Care Management: Building the Continuum* (1989) and *AIDS and Long-Term Care* (1989) and has published numerous journal articles.

John R. Kress, M.H.A., is a Senior Manager at the Association of University Programs in Health Administration (AUPHA) in Arlington, VA. He is an experienced health administrator, having worked as an executive of Family Health Care, Inc., a leading consulting firm specializing in the development and management of primary care systems and programs both domestically and abroad, and HMO development. Other affiliations have included a health planning agency, a Regional Medical Program, a cancer center development firm, and a tour as a commissioned officer in the U.S. Public Health Service. More recently, he worked with Mountain

States Health Corporation in Boise, Idaho, on a Kellogg Foundation–funded project to improve nursing home quality through the use of gerontological nurse practitioners in twelve western states. As Director of Long-Term Care and Aging for AUPHA, he directed a major grant from the Robert Wood Johnson Foundation, which added long-term care materials to the curricula of health administration programs and increased the involvement of those programs in long-term care programming. His current duties include corporate management and continuing executive education programs for executives practicing in the United States and from foreign countries. He holds a Master's degree in Health Administration from Columbia University and a B.A. degree from the City College of New York.